International travel and health

Situation as on 1 January 2011

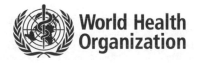
World Health
Organization

The information given in this publication is valid on the date of issue. It should be kept up to date with the notes of amendments published in the *Weekly epidemiological record* (http://www.who.int/wer).

Any comments or questions concerning this publication should be addressed to:

International Health Regulations Coordination (IHR)
Health Security and Environment (HSE)
World Health Organization
1211 Geneva 27, Switzerland
Fax: (+41) 22 791 4285
Internet access: http://www.who.int/ith

WHO Library Cataloguing-in-Publication Data

International travel and health: situation as on 1 January 2011.

    1. Communicable disease control.   2. Travel.   3. Vaccination – standards. 4. Risk factors.
    I. World Health Organization.

    ISBN 978 92 4 158046 5   (NLM classification: WA 110)
    ISSN 0254-296X

Contents

Acknowledgements

Editors: Dr Gilles Poumerol and Dr Annelies Wilder-Smith

Assistants: Ruth Anderson, Sheila Nakpil and Christèle Wantz

The following WHO personnel made contributions in their fields of expertise:

Dr Jorge Alvar
Dr Hoda Atta
Dr Bruce Aylward
Dr Mauricio Barbeschi
Dr James Bartram
Dr Eric Bertherat
Dr Gautam Biswas
Dr Léopold Blanc
Dr. Robert Bos
Dr Andrea Bosman
Dr Robert Butchart
Dr Keith Carter
Dr Claire-Lise Chaignat
Dr Yves Chartier
Dr Lester Chitsulo
Dr Eva Christophel
Dr Renu Dayal-Drager
Dr Neelam Dhingra-Kumar
Dr Philippe Duclos
Dr Chris Duncombe
Dr Mikhail Ejov
Dr Dirk Engels
Dr Rainier Escalada
Dr Socé Fall
Dr Olivier Fontaine
Dr Pierre Formenty
Dr Albis Gabrielli
Dr Biswas Gautam

Dr Bruce Gordon
Ms Anne Guilloux
Dr Max Hardiman
Dr Joachim Hombach
Dr Stéphane Hugonnet
Dr Kazuyo Ichimori
Dr Jean Jannin
Dr Georges Ki-Zerbo
Dr Rosamund Lewis
Dr Lindsay Martinez
Dr David Meddings
Dr Kamini Mendis
Dr Shanti Mendis
Dr François-Xavier Meslin
Dr Francis Ndowa
Dr Otavio Oliva
Dr Peter Olumese
Dr Fernando Otaiza
Dr Margaret Peden
Dr William Perea
Dr Pere Perez Simarro
Dr Carmen Pessoa-Da-Silva
Dr Rakesh Mani Rastogi
Dr Aafje Rietveld
Dr Pascal Ringwald
Dr Cathy Roth
Dr Lorenzo Savioli
Dr Nikky Shindo

Dr Perez Simarro
Dr Claudia Stein
Dr Rudolf Tangermann
Dr Krongthong Thimasarn
Dr Marc Van Ommeren
Dr Yvan Velez
Dr Marco Vitoria

Dr Steven Wiersma
Dr David Wood
Dr Sergio Yactayo
Dr Taghi Yasamy
Dr Morteza Zaim
Dr Ghasem Zamani

WHO gratefully acknowledges the collaboration of the International Society of Travel Medicine, the International Civil Aviation Organization, the International Air Transport Association and the International Maritime Health Association.

WHO also gratefully acknowledges the collaboration of travel medicine experts and end-users of *International travel and health* who have provided advice and information for the 2011 edition:

Dr Paul Arguin, Chief, Domestic Response Unit, Malaria Branch, Division of Parasitic Diseases, Centers for Disease Control and Prevention, Atlanta, GA, USA

Dr Karen I. Barnes, Professor, Division of Clinical Pharmacology, Department of Medicine, University of Cape Town, South Africa

Dr Ron Behrens, Department of Infectious and Tropical Diseases London School of Tropical Medicine and Hygiene, London, England

Dr Anders Björkmann, Professor, Division of Infectious Diseases, Karolinska University Hospital, Stockholm, Sweden

Dr Bjarne Bjorvatn, Professor, Centre for International Health, University of Bergen, Bergen, Norway

Dr Deborah J. Briggs, Professor, Department of Diagnostic Medicine/Pathobiology, College of Veterinary Medicine, Kansas State University, Manhattan, KS, USA

Dr Mads R. Buhl, Senior consultant in Infectious Diseases and Tropical Medicine, Aarhus University Hospital, Aarhus, Danemark

Dr Geneviève Brousse, Département des Maladies Infectieuses, Parasitaires, Tropicales et Santé Publique, Groupe Hospitalier Pitié-Salpêtrière, Paris, France

Dr Suzanne Cannegieter, Department of Clinical Epidemiology, Leiden University Medical Centre, Leiden, Netherlands

Dr Eric Caumes, Professor, Département des Maladies Infectieuses, Parasitaires, Tropicales et Santé Publique, Groupe Hospitalier Pitié-Salpêtrière, Paris, France

Dr David Chadwick, Senior Lecturer in Infectious Diseases, The James Cook University Hospital, Middlesbrough, England

Dr Charles D. Ericsson, Professor, Infectious Disease Medicine, Internal Medicine, Houston, TX, USA

Dr Anthony Evans, Chief, Aviation medicine Section, International Civil Aviation Organization, Montreal, Canada

Dr David O. Freedman, Professor of Medicine and Epidemiology, Gorgas Center for Geographic Medicine, Division of Infectious Diseases, University of Alabama at Birmingham, Birmingham, AL, USA

Mr Tom Frens, Managing Editor, Shoreland Inc., Milwaukee, WI, USA

Dr Maia Funk, Research Scientist, Division of Communicable Diseases, WHO Collaborating Centre for Travellers' Health, Institute of Social and Preventive Medicine, University of Zurich, Zurich, Switzerland

Dr Hansjakob Furrer, Professor, University Clinic for Infectious Disease, Bern University Hospital and University of Bern, Bern, Switzerland

Dr Alfons van Gompel, Associate Professor in Tropical Medicine, Institute of Tropical Medicine, Antwerpen, Belgium

Dr Peter Hackett, Altitude Research Center, University of Colorado Health Sciences Center, Aurora, CO, USA

Dr Christoph Hatz, Professor and Head of Department, Division of Communicable Diseases, Institute of Social and Preventive Medicine, University of Zurich, Zurich, Switzerland

Dr David Hill, Professor and Director, National Travel Health Network and Centre, London, England

Dr Shigeyuki Kano, Director, Department of Appropriate Technology, Development and Transfer, Research Institute, International Medical Centre of Japan, Tokyo, Japan

Dr Phyllis E. Kozarsky, Professor of Medicine/Infectious Diseases, Director, Travel and Tropical Medicine, Emory University School of Medicine, Atlanta, GA, USA

Dr Ted Lankester, Director of Health Services, InterHealth, London, England

Dr Damien Léger, Chief, Exploration et Prise en Charge des Troubles du Sommeil et de la Vigilance, Hôtel Dieu, Paris, France

Mr Graham Mapplebeck, Head of Facilitation Section, Subdivision for Maritime Security and Facilitation, International Maritime Organization, London, England

Dr Anne McCarthy, Director, Tropical Medicine and International Division of Infectious Diseases, Ottawa Hospital, General Campus, Ottawa, Canada

Dr Ziad A. Memish, Director, Gulf Cooperation Council States Center for Infection Control, King Abdulaziz Medical City, Riyadh, Saudi Arabia

Dr Marc Mendelson, Associate Professor and Head, Division of Infectious Diseases and HIV Medicine, University of Cape Town, South Africa

Dr Esperanza de Miguel García, Mental Health Department, University Hospital Virgen de las Nieves, Granada, Spain

Dr Thomas P. Monath, Kleiner Perkins Caufield & Byers, Menlo Park, CA, USA

Dr Nebojša Nikolic, Medical Centre for Occupational Health Rijeka, Faculty of Maritime Studies, University of Rijeka, Rijeka, Croatia

Dr Israel Potasman, Associate Professor, Infectious Diseases & Travel Medicine Unit, Bnai Zion Medical Center, Haifa, Israel

Dr Lars Rombo, Infektionskliniken, Eskilstuna, Sweden

Dr Patricia Schlagenhauf-Lawlor, Senior Lecturer, Research Scientist, WHO Collaborating Centre for Travellers' Health, Institute of Social and Preventive Medicine, University of Zurich, Zurich, Switzerland

Dr Pratap Sharan, Professor, Department of Psychiatry, All India Institute of Medical Sciences, New Delhi, India

Ms Natalie Shaw, Secretary of the International Shipping Federation, London, England

Dr Mark Sobsey, Professor, Environmental Sciences and Engineering, University of North Carolina at Chapel Hill, NC, USA

Dr Gerard Sonder, Head, National Coordination Center for Travellers Health Advice (LCR), Amsterdam, Netherlands

Dr Robert Steffen, Professor and Head, Division of Communicable Diseases, WHO Collaborating Centre for Travellers' Health, Institute of Social and Preventive Medicine, University of Zurich, Zurich, Switzerland

Dr Victoria Sutton, Director and Professor of Law, Center for Biodefense, Law and Public Policy, Lubbock, TX, USA

Dr Claude Thibeault, Medical Adviser, International Air Transport Association, Montreal, Canada

Dr Oyewole Tomori, Redeemer's University, Ogun State, Ikeja, Lagos State, Nigeria

Dr Jane Zuckerman, Medical Director, Academic Centre for Travel Medicine and Vaccines and WHO Collaborating Centre for Travel Medicine, Royal Free and University College Medical School, London, England

Preface

International travel is undertaken by large, and ever increasing, numbers of people for professional, social, recreational and humanitarian purposes. More people travel greater distances and at greater speed than ever before, and this upward trend looks set to continue. Travellers are thus exposed to a variety of health risks in unfamiliar environments. Most such risks, however, can be minimized by suitable precautions taken before, during and after travel. The purpose of this book is to provide guidance on measures to prevent or reduce any adverse consequences for the health of travellers.

The book is addressed primarily to medical and public health professionals who provide health advice to travellers, but it is also intended to provide guidance to travel agents and organizers, airlines and shipping companies. As far as possible, the information is presented in a form readily accessible to interested travellers and non-medical readers. For medical professionals, other sources of additional material are available and essential information is given as concisely as possible.

The book is intended to give guidance on the full range of significant health issues associated with travel. The roles of the medical profession, the travel industry and travellers themselves in avoiding health problems are recognized. The recommendations address the health risks associated with different types of travel and travellers.

While there is evidence that more traditional tourist and business travellers take appropriate prevention measures or receive proper treatment, recent immigrants who return to their home countries for the purpose of visiting friends and relatives deserve particular attention because they are at a higher risk of suffering certain health problems.

In this edition, information on yellow fever (YF) risk has been updated following the recommendations of a group of experts convened by the World Health Organization (WHO). Sao Tome and Principe, Somalia and the United Republic of Tanzania have been removed from the list of countries at risk of YF transmission

The worldwide distribution of the major infectious diseases is shown in revised maps. Vaccine-preventable disease descriptions, combined to vaccine recommendations and schedules have been rearranged and appear in alphabetical order in Chapter 6. Vaccine recommendations have been updated and chapters have been reviewed to reflect current prevention and treatment options. The main infectious diseases that pose potential health threats for travellers have been revised, as well as corresponding preventive measures and information on environmental factors that may have adverse effects on the health of travellers and well-being. The chapter on malaria provides updated information on malaria prophylaxis as well as treatment options for malaria in travellers.

The printed edition of this book is revised and published every year. The Internet version (http://www.who.int/ith) allows continuous updating and provides links to other useful information, such as: news of current disease outbreaks of international importance; useful country web links for travel and health; an interactive map for yellow fever and malaria status, requirements and recommendations; and high resolution and more precise disease distribution maps. The website also features a section on "latest updates for travellers" with recent substantial developments in travel and health.

CHAPTER 1

Health risks and precautions: general considerations

According to statistics from the World Tourism Organization, international tourist arrivals worldwide in 2009 for business, leisure and other purposes, amounted to 880 million.

Travel for leisure, recreation and holidays accounted for just over half of all international tourist arrivals (51% or 446 million arrivals). Some 15% of international tourists reported travelling for business and professional purposes and another 27% travelled for specific purposes, such as visiting friends and relatives (VFR), religious reasons and pilgrimages, health treatment, etc. Slightly over half of travellers arrived at their destination by air transport (53%) in 2009, while the remainder travelled by surface (47%) – whether by road (39%), rail (3%) or sea (5%). Over time, the share for air transport arrivals is gradually increasing.

International arrivals were expected to reach 1 billion by 2010 and 1.6 billion by 2020.

International travel can pose various risks to health, depending both on the health needs of the traveller and on the type of travel to be undertaken. Travellers may encounter sudden and significant changes in altitude, humidity, temperature and exposure to a variety of infectious diseases, which can result in illness. In addition, serious health risks may arise in areas where accommodation is of poor quality, hygiene and sanitation are inadequate, medical services are not well developed and clean water is unavailable. Accidents continue to be the most common cause of morbidity and mortality in travellers but it is also important to protect travellers against infectious diseases.

All individuals planning travel should seek advice on the potential hazards in their chosen destinations and understand how best to protect their health and minimize the risk of acquiring disease. Forward planning, appropriate preventive measures and careful precautions can protect their health and minimize the risks of accident and of acquiring disease. Although the medical profession and the travel industry can provide extensive help and advice, it remains the traveller's responsibility to seek information, to understand the risks involved and to take the necessary precautions for the journey.

1.1 Travel-related risks

Key factors in determining the risks to which a traveller may be exposed are:

— mode of transport
— destination(s)
— duration and season of travel
— purpose of travel
— standards of accommodation and food hygiene
— behaviour of the traveller
— underlying health of the traveller.

Destinations where accommodation, hygiene and sanitation, medical care and water quality are of a high standard pose relatively few serious risks to the health of travellers, except those with pre-existing illness. The same is true of business travellers and tourists visiting most major cities and tourist centres and staying in good-quality accommodation. In contrast, destinations where accommodation is of poor quality, hygiene and sanitation are inadequate, medical services do not exist and clean water is unavailable may pose serious risks for the health of travellers. This applies, for example, to personnel from emergency relief and development agencies and to tourists who venture into remote areas. In these settings, stringent precautions must be taken to avoid illness.

The epidemiology of infectious diseases in the destination country is of importance to travellers. Travellers and travel medicine practitioners should be aware of the occurrence of these diseases in the destination countries. Unforeseen natural or man-made disasters may occur; outbreaks of known or newly emerging infectious diseases are often unpredictable. New risks to international travellers may arise that are not detailed in this book but will be posted on the WHO web site (http://www.who.int), which should be regularly consulted. Similarly, up-to-date information on safety and security risks should be acquired from authoritative web sites (http://www.who.int/ith/links/national_links/en/index.html).

The mode of transport, duration of visit and the behaviour and lifestyle of the traveller are important in determining the likelihood of exposure to infectious diseases and will influence decisions on the need for certain vaccinations or antimalarial medication. The duration of visit may also determine whether the traveller is subjected to marked changes in altitude, temperature and humidity or to prolonged exposure to atmospheric pollution.

Understanding the purpose of the visit and the type of travel planned is critical in relation to the associated travel health risks. However, behaviour also plays an important role; for example, going outdoors in the evenings in a malaria-endemic area without taking precautions to avoid mosquito bites may result in the traveller becoming infected with malaria. Exposure to insects, rodents or other animals, infectious agents and contaminated food and water, combined with the absence of appropriate medical facilities, makes travel in many remote regions particularly hazardous.

Whatever their destination or mode of travel, it is important that travellers should be aware of the risk of accidents under the influence of alcohol or drugs and, mainly, in relation to road transport or the practice of sports.

1.2 Medical consultation before travel

Travellers intending to visit a destination in a developing country should consult a travel medicine clinic or medical practitioner before the journey. This consultation should take place at least 4–8 weeks before the journey and preferably earlier if long-term travel or overseas work is envisaged. However, last-minute travellers can also benefit from a medical consultation, even as late as the day of travel. The consultation will include information about the most important health risks (including traffic accidents), and determine the need for any vaccinations and/or antimalarial medication and identify any other medical items that the traveller may require. A basic medical kit will be prescribed or provided, supplemented as appropriate to meet individual needs.

Dental and gynaecological check-ups are advisable before prolonged travel to developing countries or to remote areas. This is particularly important for people with chronic or recurrent dental or gynaecological/obstetric diseases or problems. Travellers with underlying medical problems are strongly advised to consult a travel medicine clinic or medical practitioner to ensure that their potentially complex travel health needs are met. All travellers should be strongly advised to seek comprehensive travel insurance.

1.3 Assessment of health risks associated with travel

Medical advisers base their recommendations, including those for vaccinations and other medication, on an assessment of risk for the individual traveller, which takes into account the likelihood of acquiring a disease and how serious this might be for the person concerned. Key elements of this risk assessment are the pre-travel health status of the traveller, destination(s), duration and purpose of travel, the mode of transport, standards of accommodation and food hygiene, and risk behaviour while travelling.

3

For each disease being considered, an assessment is also made of:

— availability of appropriate medical services in the destination, prophylaxis, emergency treatment packs, self-treatment kits (e.g. a travellers' diarrhoea kit);
— any associated public health risks (e.g. the risk of infecting others).

Collecting the information required to make a risk assessment involves detailed questioning of the traveller. A checklist or protocol is useful to ensure that all relevant information is obtained and recorded. The traveller should be provided with a personal record of the vaccinations given (patient-retained record) including, for example, intramuscular administration of rabies vaccine, as vaccinations are often administered at different centres. A model checklist, reproducible for individual travellers, is provided at the end of this chapter.

1.4 Medical kit and toilet items

Sufficient medical supplies should be carried to meet foreseeable needs for the duration of the trip.

A medical kit should be carried for all destinations where there may be significant health risks, particularly those in developing countries and/or where the local availability of specific medications is uncertain. This kit will include basic medicines to treat common ailments, first-aid articles, and any other special medical items, such as syringes and needles (to minimize exposure to bloodborne viruses), that may be needed and can in some cases be used by the individual traveller.

Certain categories of prescription medicine or special medical item should be carried together with a medical attestation on letterhead, signed by a physician, certifying that the traveller requires the medication or the items for a medical condition. Some countries require that this attestation be signed not only by a physician but also by the national health administration.

Toilet items should also be carried in sufficient quantity for the entire visit unless their availability at the travel destination is assured. These will include items for dental care, eye care (including contact lenses), skin care and personal hygiene.

Contents of a basic medical kit

First-aid items:

— adhesive tape
— antiseptic wound cleanser or alkaline soap
— bandages

— scissors
— safety pins
— emollient (lubricant) eye drops
— insect repellent
— insect bite treatment
— antihistamine tablets
— nasal decongestant
— oral rehydration salts
— simple analgesic (e.g. paracetamol)
— sterile dressing
— clinical thermometer
— sunscreen
— earplugs
— tweezers
— adhesive strips to close small wounds.

Additional items according to destination and individual needs:

— antidiarrhoeal medication (to include an antisecretory agent, an antimotility drug, oral rehydration salts, with appropriate written instructions regarding their use)
— antibiotics targeting the most frequent infections in travellers (e.g. travellers' diarrhoea, and infections of skin and soft-tissue, respiratory tract and urinary tract)
— antibacterial ointment
— antifungal powder
— antimalarial medication
— mosquito net and insecticide to treat fabrics (clothes, nets, curtains)
— adequate supplies of condoms and oral contraceptives
— medication for pre-existing medical conditions
— sterile syringes and needles
— water disinfectant
— spare eyeglasses and/or spare contact lenses (and solution)
— other items to meet foreseeable needs, according to the destination and duration of the visit.

1.5 Travellers with pre-existing medical conditions and special needs

Health risks associated with travel are greater for certain groups of travellers, including infants and young children, pregnant women, the elderly, the disabled, the immunocompromised and those who have pre-existing health problems. Health risks may also vary depending on the purpose of travel, such as travel to visit friends and relatives or for religious purposes/pilgrimages (Chapter 9), for relief work or for business. All of these travellers need both general medical advice and specific travel health advice, including special precautions. Travellers should be advised to seek information about the available medical services at their travel destinations.

1.5.1 Age

Air travel may cause discomfort to infants as a result of changes in cabin air pressure and is contraindicated for infants less than 48 h old. Infants and young children are particularly sensitive to sudden changes in altitude and to ultraviolet radiation. They have special needs with regard to vaccinations and antimalarial precautions (Chapters 6 and 7). They become dehydrated more easily than adults in the event of inadequate fluid intake or loss of fluid as a result of diarrhoea and can be overcome by dehydration within a few hours. They are also more susceptible to infectious diseases.

Advanced age is not necessarily a contraindication for travel if the general health status is good. Elderly people should seek medical advice before planning long-distance travel.

1.5.2 Pregnancy

Travel is not generally contraindicated during pregnancy until close to the expected date of delivery, provided that the pregnancy is uncomplicated and the woman's health is good. It is safest for pregnant women to travel during the second trimester. Airlines impose some travel restrictions in late pregnancy and in the neonatal period (Chapter 2). It is advisable for travellers to check any restrictions directly with the relevant airline.

There are some restrictions on vaccination during pregnancy: specific information is provided in Chapter 6.

Pregnant women risk serious complications if they contract malaria or viral hepatitis E. Travel to areas endemic for these diseases should be avoided during pregnancy if at all possible. Specific recommendations for the use of antimalarial drugs during pregnancy are given in Chapter 7.

Medication of any type during pregnancy should be taken only in accordance with medical advice.

Travel to sleeping altitudes over 3000 m (Chapter 3) or to remote areas is not advisable during pregnancy.

1.5.3 Disability

Physical disability is not usually a contraindication for travel if the general health status of the traveller is good. Airlines have regulations concerning travel for disabled passengers who need to be accompanied (Chapter 2). Information should be obtained from the relevant airline well in advance of the intended travel.

1.5.4 Pre-existing illness

People suffering from underlying chronic illnesses should seek medical advice before planning a journey. Conditions that increase health risks during travel include:

— cardiovascular disorders
— chronic hepatitis
— chronic inflammatory bowel disease
— chronic renal disease requiring dialysis
— chronic respiratory diseases
— diabetes mellitus
— epilepsy
— immunosuppression due to medication or to HIV infection
— previous thromboembolic disease
— severe anaemia
— severe mental disorders
— any chronic condition requiring frequent medical intervention
— transplantation
— chronic haematological conditions.

Travellers with a chronic illness should carry all necessary medication and medical items for the entire duration of the journey. All medications, especially prescription medications, should be packed in carry-on luggage, in their original containers with clear labels. A duplicate supply carried in the checked luggage is a safety precaution against loss or theft. With heightened airline security, sharp objects and liquids in quantities of more than 100 ml will have to remain in checked luggage.

Travellers should carry the name and contact details of their physician on their person with other travel documents, together with information about the medical condition and treatment, and details of medication (generic drug names included)

7

and prescribed doses. This information should also be stored electronically for remote retrieval, e.g. on a secure database. A physician's attestation should also be carried, certifying the necessity for any drugs or other medical items (e.g. syringes) carried by the traveller that may be questioned by customs officials and/ or security personnel.

1.6 Insurance for travellers

Travellers are strongly advised to travel with comprehensive travel insurance as a matter of routine and to declare any underlying health conditions. Travellers should be aware that medical care abroad is often available only at private medical facilities and may be costly. In places where good-quality medical care is not readily available, travellers may need to be repatriated in case of accident or illness. If death occurs abroad, repatriation of the body can be extremely expensive and may be difficult to arrange. Travellers are advised (i) to seek information about possible reciprocal health-care agreements between the country of residence and the destination country, and (ii) to obtain special travellers' health insurance for destinations where health risks are significant and medical care is expensive or not readily available. This health insurance should include coverage for changes to the itinerary, emergency repatriation for health reasons, hospitalization, medical care in case of illness or accident and repatriation of the body in case of death. Travellers should discuss with the parties concerned any issues or claims as they happen and not upon return from the trip.

Travel agents and tour operators usually provide information about travellers' health insurance. It should be noted that some countries now require proof of adequate health insurance as a condition for entry. Moreover, some travel insurers require proof of immunizations and/or malaria prophylaxis as a condition of their approval for treatment or repatriation. Travellers should know the procedures to follow to obtain assistance and reimbursement. A copy of the insurance certificate and contact details should be carried with other travel documents in the hand luggage.

1.7 Role of travel industry professionals

Tour operators, travel agents, airline and shipping companies each have an important responsibility to safeguard the health of travellers. It is in the interests of the travel industry that travellers have the fewest possible problems when travelling to, and visiting, foreign countries. Contact with travellers before the journey provides a unique opportunity to inform them of the situation in each of the countries they are visiting. The travel agent or tour operator should provide travellers with the following health-related guidance (or the tools to access this information):

- Advise travellers to consult a travel medicine clinic or medical practitioner as soon as possible after planning a trip to any destination where significant health risks may be foreseen, particularly those in developing countries, preferably 4–8 weeks before departure.

- Advise last-minute travellers to visit to a travel medicine clinic or medical practitioner, which can be done even on the day before departure.

- Inform travellers of any particular hazards to personal safety and security presented by the destination and suggest appropriate precautions including checking authoritative web sites (http://www.who.int/ith/links/national_links/en/index.html) on a regular basis.

- Encourage travellers to take out comprehensive travellers' health insurance and provide information on available policies.

- Inform travellers of the procedures for obtaining assistance and reimbursement, particularly if the insurance policy is arranged by the travel agent or company.

- Provide information on:
  - mandatory vaccination requirements for yellow fever;
  - the need for malaria precautions at the travel destination;
  - the existence of other important health hazards at the travel destination;
  - the presence or absence of good-quality medical facilities at the travel destination.

1.8 Responsibility of the traveller

Travellers can obtain a great deal of information and advice from medical and travel industry professionals to help prevent health problems while abroad. However, travellers are responsible for their health and well-being while travelling and on their return, as well as for preventing the transmission of communicable diseases to others. The following are the main responsibilities of the traveller:

- the decision to travel;
- recognizing and accepting any risks involved;
- seeking health advice in good time, preferably 4–8 weeks before travel;
- complying with recommended vaccinations and other prescribed medication and health measures;
- careful planning before departure;

- carrying a medical kit and understanding its use;
- obtaining adequate insurance cover;
- taking health precautions before, during and after the journey;
- obtaining a physician's attestation pertaining to any prescription medicines, syringes, etc. being carried;
- the health and well-being of accompanying children;
- taking precautions to avoid transmitting any infectious disease to others during and after travel;
- full reporting to a medical professional of any illness on return, including information about all recent travel;
- being respectful of the host country and its population;
- practising responsible sexual behaviour and avoiding unprotected sexual contact.

A model checklist for use by travellers, indicating steps to be taken before the journey, is provided at the end of the chapter.

1.9 Medical examination after travel

Travellers are advised to have a medical examination on their return if they:

- suffer from a chronic disease, such as cardiovascular disease, diabetes mellitus, or chronic respiratory disease or have been taking anticoagulants;
- experience illness in the weeks following their return home, particularly if fever, persistent diarrhoea, vomiting, jaundice, urinary disorders, skin disease or genital infection occurs;
- they received treatment for malaria while travelling;
- may have been exposed to a serious infectious disease while travelling;
- have spent more than 3 months in a developing country.

Travellers should provide medical personnel with information on recent travel, including destination, and purpose and duration of visit. Frequent travellers should give details of all journeys that have taken place in the preceding weeks and months including pre-travel vaccinations received and malaria chemoprophylaxis taken.

Note. Fever after returning from a malaria-endemic area is a medical emergency and travellers who develop fever should seek medical attention immediately, explaining that they may have contracted malaria.

Further reading

Keystone JS et al., eds. *Travel medicine*, 2nd ed. London, Elsevier, 2008.

UNWTO tourism highlights. Madrid, World Tourism Organization, 2009 (available at http://www.unwto.org/facts/eng/highlights.htm).

Steffen R, Dupont HL, Wilder-Smith A, eds. *Manual of travel medicine and health*, 2nd ed. London, BC Decker, 2007.

Zuckerman JN, ed. *Principles and practice of travel medicine*. Chichester, Wiley, 2001 (2nd edition in press).

Checklist for the traveller

Obtain information on local conditions

Depending on destination

- risks related to the area (urban or rural)
- type of accommodation (hotel, camping)
- length of stay
- altitude
- security problems (e.g. conflict)
- availability of medical facilities.

Prevention

Vaccination. Contact the nearest travel medicine centre or a physician as early as possible, preferably 4–8 weeks before departure.

Malaria. Request information on malaria risk, prevention of mosquito bites, possible need for appropriate preventive medication and emergency reserves; pack a bednet and insect repellent.

Food hygiene. Eat only thoroughly cooked food and drink only bottled or packaged cold drinks, ensuring that the seal has not been broken. Boil drinking-water if safety is doubtful. If boiling is not possible, a certified well-maintained filter and/or disinfectant agent can be used.

Specific local diseases. Consult the appropriate sections of this book as well as http://www.who.int and authoritative web sites (http://www.who.int/ith/links/national_links/en/index.html).

Be aware of accidents related to

- traffic (obtain and carry a card showing blood group before departure)
- animals (beware of venomous marine or land creatures and other animals that may be rabid)
- allergies (wear a medical alert bracelet)
- sun (pack sunglasses and sunscreen)
- sport

Get the following check-ups

- medical — obtain prescriptions for medication according to length of stay, and obtain advice from your physician on assembling a suitable medical kit
- dental
- other according to specific conditions (e.g. pregnancy, diabetes)

Insurance

Purchase medical insurance with appropriate cover abroad, i.e. accident, sickness, medical repatriation.

Pre-departure travel health record

Surname:	First name(s):
Date of birth:	Country of current residence:

Purpose of travel: ☐ Tourist   ☐ Business   ☐ NGO and other traveller categorie

☐ Visiting friends and/or relatives

Special activities: ☐ Accommodation: e.g. camping, bivouac

☐ Sports: e.g. diving, hunting, high-altitude trekking

☐ Adventure: e.g. bungee, jumping, white-water rafting

Date of departure and length of stay:

Places to be visited

Country	Town	Rural area		Dates	
		Yes	No	From	to
		Yes	No	From	to
		Yes	No	From	to
		Yes	No	From	to
		Yes	No	From	to

Medical history

Vaccination record including details of vaccination received to date:

Current state of health:

Chronic illnesses:

Recent or current medical treatment, including current medications:

Allergies (e.g. eggs, antibiotics, sulfonamides):

For women: ☐ Current pregnancy

☐ Pregnancy likely within 3 months

☐ Currently breastfeeding

History of anxiety or depression:

☐ If yes, treatment prescribed (specify):

Neurological disorders (e.g. epilepsy, multiple sclerosis):

Cardiovascular disorders (e.g. thrombosis, use of pacemaker):

CHAPTER 2

Mode of travel: health considerations

Travel by air and by sea exposes passengers to a number of factors that may have an impact on health. In this chapter, technical terms have been used sparingly in order to facilitate use by a wide readership. Medical professionals needing more detailed information are referred to the web site of the Aerospace Medical Association (http://www.asma.org) and the web site of the International Maritime Health Association (http://www.imha.net/).

2.1 Travel by air

The volume of air traffic has continued to rise over the years and "frequent flyers" now make up a substantial proportion of the travelling public. The number of long-haul flights has increased. According to the International Civil Aviation Organization, passenger traffic is projected to double between 2006 and 2020.

Air travel, particularly over long distances, exposes passengers to a number of factors that may have an effect on their health and well-being. Travellers with pre-existing health problems and those receiving medical care are more likely to be affected and should consult their doctor or a travel medicine clinic in good time before travelling. Health risks associated with air travel can be minimized if the traveller plans carefully and takes some simple precautions before, during and after the flight. An explanation of the various factors that may affect the health and well-being of air travellers follows.

2.1.1 Cabin air pressure

Although aircraft cabins are pressurized, cabin air pressure at cruising altitude is lower than air pressure at sea level. At typical cruising altitudes in the range 11 000–12 200 m (36 000–40 000 feet), air pressure in the cabin is equivalent to the outside air pressure at 1800–2400 m (6000–8000 feet) above sea level. As a consequence, less oxygen is taken up by the blood (hypoxia) and gases within the body expand. The effects of reduced cabin air pressure are usually well tolerated by healthy passengers.

Oxygen and hypoxia

Cabin air contains ample oxygen for healthy passengers and crew. However, because cabin air pressure is relatively low, the amount of oxygen carried in the blood is reduced compared with that at sea level. Passengers with certain medical conditions, particularly heart and lung diseases and blood disorders such as anaemia (in particular sickle-cell anaemia), may not tolerate this reduced oxygen level (hypoxia) very well. Some of these passengers are able to travel safely if arrangements are made with the airline for the provision of an additional oxygen supply during flight. However, because regulations and practices differ from country to country and between airlines, it is strongly recommended that these travellers, especially those wishing to carry their own oxygen, contact the airline early in their travel plans. An additional charge is often levied on passengers who require supplemental oxygen to be provided by the airline.

Gas expansion

As the aircraft climbs in altitude after take-off, the decreasing cabin air pressure causes gases to expand. Similarly, as the aircraft descends in altitude before landing, the increasing pressure in the cabin causes gases to contract. These changes may have effects where air is trapped in the body.

Passengers often experience a "popping" sensation in the ears caused by air escaping from the middle ear and the sinuses during the aircraft's climb. This is not usually considered a problem. As the aircraft descends in altitude prior to landing, air must flow back into the middle ear and sinuses in order to equalize pressure. If this does not happen, the ears or sinuses may feel as if they are blocked and pain can result. Swallowing, chewing or yawning ("clearing the ears") will usually relieve any discomfort. As soon as it is recognized that the problem will not resolve itself using these methods, a short forceful expiration against a pinched nose and closed mouth (Valsalva manoeuvre) should be tried and will usually help. For infants, feeding or giving a pacifier (dummy) to stimulate swallowing may reduce the symptoms.

Individuals with ear, nose and sinus infections should avoid flying because pain and injury may result from the inability to equalize pressure differences. If travel cannot be avoided, the use of decongestant nasal drops shortly before the flight and again before descent may be helpful.

As the aircraft climbs, expansion of gas in the abdomen can cause discomfort, although this is usually mild.

Some forms of surgery (e.g. abdominal surgery) and other medical treatments or tests (e.g. treatment for a detached retina) may introduce air or other gases into a body cavity. Travellers who have recently undergone such procedures should ask a travel medicine physician or their treating physician how long they should wait before undertaking air travel.

2.1.2 Cabin humidity and dehydration

The humidity in aircraft cabins is low, usually less than 20% (humidity in the home is normally over 30%). Low humidity may cause skin dryness and discomfort to the eyes, mouth and nose but presents no risk to health. Use skin moisturizing lotion or a saline nasal spray to moisturize the nasal passages. Wearing eyeglasses rather than contact lenses can relieve or prevent discomfort to the eyes. The available evidence has not shown low humidity to cause internal dehydration and there is no need to drink more than usual. However, since caffeine and alcohol have a diuretic effect (causing more urine to be produced), it is wise to limit consumption of such beverages during long flights.

2.1.3 Ozone

Ozone is a form of oxygen that occurs in the upper atmosphere and may enter the aircraft cabin together with the fresh-air supply. In older aircraft, it was found that the levels of ozone in cabin air could sometimes lead to irritation of the lungs, eyes and nasal tissues. Ozone is broken down by heat and a significant amount of ozone is removed by the engine compressors (which compress and heat the air) that provide pressurized air for the cabin. In addition, most modern long-haul jet aircraft are fitted with equipment (catalytic converters) that breaks down any remaining ozone.

2.1.4 Cosmic radiation

Cosmic radiation is made up of radiation that comes from the sun and from outer space. The Earth's atmosphere and magnetic field are natural shields and cosmic radiation levels are therefore lower at lower altitudes. The Earth's population is continually exposed to natural background radiation from soil, rock and building materials as well as from cosmic radiation that reaches the Earth's surface.

Cosmic radiation is more intense over polar regions than over the equator because of the shape of the Earth's magnetic field and the "flattening" of the atmosphere over the poles. Although cosmic radiation levels are higher at aircraft cruising altitudes than at sea level, research has not shown any significant health effects for aircraft passengers or crew.

2.1.5 Motion sickness

Except in the case of severe turbulence, travellers by air rarely suffer from motion sickness. Those who do suffer should request a seat in the mid-section of the cabin where movements are less pronounced, and keep the motion sickness bag, provided at each seat, readily accessible. They should also consult their doctor or travel medicine physician about medication that can be taken before flying to help prevent problems, and should avoid drinking alcohol during the flight and for 24 h beforehand.

2.1.6 Immobility, circulatory problems and deep vein thrombosis (DVT)

Contraction of muscles is an important factor in helping to keep blood flowing through the veins, particularly in the legs. Prolonged immobility, especially when seated, can lead to pooling of blood in the legs, which in turn may cause swelling, stiffness and discomfort.

It is known that immobility is one of the factors that may lead to the development of a blood clot in a deep vein – so-called "deep vein thrombosis" or DVT. Research has shown that DVT can occur as a result of prolonged immobility, for instance during long-distance travel, whether by car, bus, train or air. WHO set up a major research study, WHO Research Into Global Hazards of Travel (WRIGHT), in order to establish whether the risk of venous thromboembolism is increased by air travel, to determine the magnitude of the risk and the effect of other factors on the risk, and to study the effect of preventive measures. The findings of the epidemiological studies indicate that the risk of venous thromboembolism is increased 2- to 3-fold after long-haul flights (>4 h) and also with other forms of travel involving prolonged seated immobility. The risk increases with the duration of travel and with multiple flights within a short period. In absolute terms, an average of 1 passenger in 6000 will suffer from venous thromboembolism after a long-haul flight.

In most cases of DVT, the clots are small and do not cause any symptoms. The body is able to gradually break down the clots and there are no long-term effects. Larger clots may cause symptoms such as swelling of the leg, tenderness, soreness and pain. Occasionally a piece of a clot may break off and travel with the bloodstream, to become lodged in the lungs. This is known as pulmonary embolism and may cause chest pain, shortness of breath and, in severe cases, sudden death. This can occur many hours or even days after the formation of the clot in the leg.

The risk of developing DVT when travelling is increased in the presence of other risk factors, including:

- previous DVT or pulmonary embolism
- history of DVT or pulmonary embolism in a close family member
- use of oestrogen therapy – oral contraceptives ("the pill") or hormone-replacement therapy (HRT)
- pregnancy
- recent surgery or trauma, particularly to the abdomen, pelvic region or legs
- cancer
- obesity
- some inherited blood-clotting abnormalities.

DVT occurs more commonly in older people. Some researchers have suggested that there may be a risk from smoking and from varicose veins.

It is advisable for people with one or more of these risk factors to seek specific medical advice from their doctor or a travel medicine clinic in good time before embarking on a flight of four or more hours.

Precautions

The benefits of most recommended precautionary measures in travellers at particular risk for DVT are unproven and some might even result in harm. Further studies to identify effective preventive measures are ongoing. However, some general advice for such passengers is given here.

- Moving around the cabin during long flights will help to reduce any period of prolonged immobility, although this may not always be possible. Moreover, any potential health benefits must be balanced against the risk of injury if the aircraft were to experience sudden turbulence. A regular trip to the bathroom, e.g. every 2–3 h, is a reasonable measure.

- Many airlines provide helpful advice on exercises that can be carried out in the seat during flight. Exercise of the calf muscles can stimulate the circulation, alleviate discomfort, fatigue and stiffness, and may reduce the risk of developing DVT.

- Hand luggage should not be placed where it restricts movement of the legs and feet, and clothing should be loose and comfortable.

- In view of the clear risk of significant side effects and absence of clear evidence of benefit, passengers are advised not to use aspirin specifically for the prevention of travel-related DVT.

- Those travellers at greatest risk of developing DVT may be prescribed specific treatments and should consult their doctor for further advice.

2.1.7 Diving

Divers should avoid flying soon after diving because of the risk that the reduced cabin pressure may lead to decompression sickness (more commonly called "the bends"). It is recommended that they do not fly until at least 12 h after the last dive; this period should be extended to 24 h after multiple dives or after diving that requires decompression stops during ascent to the surface. Travellers should seek specialist advice from diving schools. Divers Alert Network is an excellent source of information with a good Frequently Asked Questions section (http://www.diversalertnetwork.org/medical/faq/Default.aspx) as well as an emergency hotline number.

2.1.8 Jet lag

Jet lag is the term used for the symptoms caused by the disruption of the body's "internal clock" and the approximate 24-h (circadian) rhythms it controls. Disruption occurs when crossing multiple time zones, i.e. when flying east to west or west to east. Jet lag may lead to indigestion and disturbance of bowel function, general malaise, daytime sleepiness, difficulty in sleeping at night, and reduced physical and mental performance. Its effects are often combined with tiredness caused by the journey itself. Jet lag symptoms gradually wear off as the body adapts to the new time zone.

Jet lag cannot be prevented but there are ways of reducing its effects (see below). Travellers who take medication according to a strict timetable (e.g. insulin, oral contraceptives) should seek medical advice from their doctor or a travel medicine clinic before their journey.

General measures to reduce the effects of jet lag

- Be as well rested as possible before departure, and use any opportunity to rest during medium to long-haul flights. Even short naps (less than 40 min) can be helpful.

- Eat light meals and limit consumption of alcohol. Alcohol increases urine output, with the result that sleep may be disturbed by the need to urinate. While it can accelerate the onset of sleep, alcohol impairs the quality of sleep, making it less restful. The after-effects of excessive consumption of alcohol ("hangover") can exacerbate the effects of jet lag and travel fatigue. Alcohol should therefore be consumed in moderation, if at all, before and during the flight. Caffeine should be limited to normal amounts and avoided within 4–6 h of an expected period of sleep. If coffee is drunk during the daytime, small amounts every 2 h or so are preferable to a single large cup.

- At destination, try to create the right conditions when preparing for sleep and get as much sleep in as normal in the 24 h after arrival. A minimum block of 4 h sleep during the local night – known as "anchor sleep" – is thought to be necessary to allow the body's internal clock to adapt to the new time zone. If possible, make up the total sleep time by taking naps during the day in response to feelings of sleepiness. When taking a nap during the day, eyeshades and earplugs may help. Exercise during the day may help to promote a good night's sleep, but avoid strenuous exercise within 2 h of trying to sleep.

- The cycle of light and dark is one of the most important factors in setting the body's internal clock. A well-timed exposure to daylight, preferably bright sunlight, at the destination will usually help adaptation. When flying west, exposure to daylight in the evening and avoidance in the morning (e.g. by using eye shades or dark glasses) may be helpful; flying east, exposure to light in the morning and avoidance in the evening are to be recommended.

- Short-acting sleeping pills may be helpful. They should be used only in accordance with medical advice and should not normally be taken during the flight, as they may increase immobility and therefore the risk of developing DVT.

- Melatonin is available in some countries. It is normally sold as a food supplement and therefore is not subject to the same strict control as medications (for example, it has not been approved for use as a medication in the United States, but can be sold as a food supplement). The timing and effective dosage of melatonin have not been fully evaluated and its side-effects, particularly in long-term use, are unknown. Moreover, manufacturing methods are not standardized: the dose per tablet can vary considerably and some harmful compounds may be present. For these reasons, melatonin cannot be recommended.

- Trying to adjust to local time for short trips of up to 2–3 days may not be the best coping strategy, because the body clock may not have an opportunity to synchronize to the new time zone, and re-synchronization to the home time zone may be delayed after the return flight. If in doubt, seek specialist travel medicine advice.

- Individuals react in different ways to time zone changes. Frequent flyers should learn how their own bodies respond and adopt habits accordingly. Advice from a travel medicine clinic may help in formulating an effective coping strategy.

2.1.9 Psychological aspects

Stress, fear of flying (flight phobia), air rage and other psychological aspects of air travel are detailed in Chapter 10.

2.1.10 Travellers with medical conditions or special needs

Airlines have the right to refuse to carry passengers with conditions that may worsen, or have serious consequences, during the flight. They may require medical clearance from their medical department/adviser if there is an indication that a passenger could be suffering from any disease or physical or mental condition that:

— may be considered a potential hazard to the safety of the aircraft;
— adversely affects the welfare and comfort of the other passengers and/or crew members;
— requires medical attention and/or special equipment during the flight;
— may be aggravated by the flight.

If cabin crew suspect before departure that a passenger may be ill, the aircraft's captain will be informed and a decision taken as to whether the passenger is fit to travel, needs medical attention or presents a danger to other passengers and crew or to the safety of the aircraft.

Although this chapter provides some general guidelines on conditions that may require medical clearance in advance, airline policies vary and requirements should always be checked at the time of, or before, booking the flight. A good place to find information is often the airline's own web site.

Infants
A fit and healthy baby can travel by air 48 h after birth, but it is preferable to wait until the age of 7 days. Until their organs have developed properly and stabilized, premature babies should always undergo a medical clearance before travelling by air. Changes in cabin air pressure may upset infants; this can be helped by feeding or giving a pacifier to stimulate swallowing.

Pregnant women
Pregnant women can normally travel safely by air, but most airlines restrict travel in late pregnancy. Typical guidelines for a woman with an uncomplicated pregnancy are:

— after the 28th week of pregnancy, a letter from a doctor or midwife should be carried, confirming the expected date of delivery and that the pregnancy is normal;
— for single pregnancies, flying is permitted up to the end of the 36th week;
— for multiple pregnancies, flying is permitted up to the end of the 32nd week.

Each case of complicated pregnancy requires medical clearance.

Pre-existing illness

Most people with medical conditions are able to travel safely by air, provided that necessary precautions, such as the need for additional oxygen supply, are considered in advance.

Those who have underlying health problems such as cancer, heart or lung disease, anaemia and diabetes, who are on any form of regular medication or treatment, who have recently had surgery or been in hospital, or who are concerned about their fitness to travel for any other reason should consult their doctor or a travel medicine clinic before deciding to travel by air.

Medication that may be required during the journey, or soon after arrival, should be carried in the hand luggage. It is also advisable to carry a copy of the prescription in case the medication is lost, additional supplies are needed or security checks require proof of purpose (Chapter 1).

Frequent travellers with medical conditions

A frequent traveller who has a permanent and stable underlying health problem may obtain a frequent traveller's medical card (or equivalent) from the medical or reservation department of many airlines. This card is accepted, under specified conditions, as proof of medical clearance and for identification of the holder's medical condition.

Dental/oral surgery

Recent dental procedures such as fillings are not usually a contraindication to flying. However, unfinished root canal treatment and dental abscesses are reasons for caution, and it is recommended that individuals seek advice with regard to travel plans from the surgeon or dental practitioner most familiar with their case.

Security issues

Security checks can cause concerns for travellers who have been fitted with metal devices such as artificial joints, pacemakers or internal automatic defibrillators. Some pacemakers may be affected by modern security screening equipment and any traveller with a pacemaker should carry a letter from their doctor.

Smokers

Almost all airlines now ban smoking on board. Some smokers may find this stressful, particularly during long flights, and should discuss the issue with a doctor before travelling. Nicotine replacement patches or chewing gum containing nicotine may be helpful during the flight and the use of other medication or techniques may also be considered.

Travellers with disabilities

A physical disability is not usually a contraindication for travel. A passenger who is unable to look after his or her own needs during the flight (including use of the toilet and transfer from wheelchair to seat and vice versa) will need to be accompanied by an escort able to provide all necessary assistance. The cabin crew are generally not permitted to provide such assistance and a traveller who requires it but does not have a suitable escort may not be permitted to travel. Travellers confined to wheelchairs should be advised against deliberately restricting fluid intake before or during travel as a means of avoiding use of the toilet during flights, as this may be detrimental to overall health.

Airlines have regulations on conditions of travel for passengers with disabilities. Disabled passengers should contact airlines for guidance in advance of travel; the airlines' own web sites often give useful information.

2.1.11 Transmission of communicable diseases on aircraft

Research has shown that there is very little risk of any communicable disease being transmitted on board an aircraft.

The quality of aircraft cabin air is carefully controlled. Ventilation rates provide a total change of air 20–30 times per hour. Most modern aircraft have recirculation systems, which recycle up to 50% of cabin air. The recirculated air is usually passed through HEPA (high-efficiency particulate air) filters, of the type used in hospital operating theatres and intensive care units, which trap dust particles, bacteria, fungi and viruses.

Transmission of infection may occur between passengers who are seated in the same area of an aircraft, usually as a result of the infected individual coughing or sneezing or by touch (direct contact or contact with the same parts of the aircraft cabin and furnishings that other passengers touch). This is no different from any other situation in which people are close to each other, such as on a train or bus or in a theatre. Highly contagious conditions, such as influenza, are more likely to be spread to other passengers in situations where the aircraft ventilation system is not operating. An auxiliary power unit is normally used to provide ventilation when the aircraft is on the ground, before the main engines are started, but occasionally this is not operated for environmental (noise) or technical reasons. In such cases, when associated with a prolonged delay, passengers may be temporarily disembarked.

Transmission of tuberculosis (TB) on board commercial aircraft during long-haul flights was reported during the 1980s, but no case of active TB disease resulting from exposure on board has been identified subsequently. Nevertheless, increasing air travel and the emergence of drug-resistant TB require continuing vigilance to avoid the spread of infection during air travel. Further information on TB and air travel may be found in the 2008 edition of the WHO publication *Tuberculosis and air travel: guidelines for prevention and control.*

During the outbreak of severe acute respiratory syndrome (SARS) in 2003, the risk of transmission of the disease in aircraft was found to be very low.

To minimize the risk of passing on infections, travellers who are unwell, particularly if they have a fever, should delay their journey until they have recovered. Individuals with a known active communicable disease should not travel by air. Airlines may deny boarding to passengers who appear to be infected with a communicable disease.

2.1.12 Aircraft disinsection

Many countries require disinsection of aircraft (to kill insects) arriving from countries where diseases that are spread by insects, such as malaria and yellow fever, occur. There have been a number of cases of malaria affecting individuals who live or work in the vicinity of airports in countries where malaria is not present, thought to be due to the escape of malaria-carrying mosquitoes transported on aircraft. Some countries, e.g. Australia and New Zealand, routinely carry out disinsection to prevent the inadvertent introduction of species that may harm their agriculture.

Disinsection is a public health measure that is mandated by the International Health Regulations (Annex 2). It involves treatment of the interior of the aircraft with insecticides specified by WHO. The different procedures currently in use are as follows:

— treatment of the interior of the aircraft using a quick-acting insecticide spray immediately before take-off, with the passengers on board;
— treatment of the interior of the aircraft on the ground before passengers come on board, using a residual-insecticide aerosol, plus additional in-flight treatment with a quick-acting spray shortly before landing;
— regular application of a residual insecticide to all internal surfaces of the aircraft, except those in food preparation areas.

Passengers are sometimes concerned about their exposure to insecticide sprays during air travel, and some have reported feeling unwell after spraying of aircraft for disinsection. However, WHO has found no evidence that the specified insecticide sprays are harmful to human health when used as recommended.

2.1.13 Medical assistance on board

Airlines are required to provide minimum levels of medical equipment on aircraft and to train all cabin crew in first aid. The equipment carried varies, with many airlines carrying more than the minimum level of equipment required by regulations. Equipment carried on a typical international flight would include:

— one or more first-aid kits, to be used by the crew;
— a medical kit, normally to be used by a doctor or other qualified person, to treat in-flight medical emergencies.

An automated external defibrillator (AED), to be used by the crew in case of cardiac arrest, is also carried by several airlines.

Cabin crew are trained in the use of first-aid equipment and in carrying out first-aid and resuscitation procedures. They are usually also trained to recognize a range of medical conditions that may cause emergencies on board and to act appropriately to manage these.

In addition, many airlines have facilities to enable crew to contact a medical expert at a ground-based response centre for advice on how to manage in-flight medical emergencies.

2.1.14 Contraindications to air travel

Travel by air is normally contraindicated in the following cases:

● Infants less than 48 h old.

● Women after the 36th week of pregnancy (32nd week for multiple pregnancies).

● Those suffering from:
— angina pectoris or chest pain at rest;
— any active communicable disease;
— decompression sickness after diving;
— increased intracranial pressure due to haemorrhage, trauma or infection;
— infections of the sinuses or of the ear and nose, particularly if the Eustachian tube is blocked;

- recent myocardial infarction and stroke (elapsed time since the event depending on severity of illness and duration of travel);
- recent surgery or injury where trapped air or gas may be present, especially abdominal trauma and gastrointestinal surgery, craniofacial and ocular injuries, brain operations, and eye operations involving penetration of the eyeball;
- severe chronic respiratory disease, breathlessness at rest, or unresolved pneumothorax;
- sickle-cell anaemia;
- psychotic illness, except when fully controlled.

The above list is not comprehensive, and fitness for travel should be decided on a case-by-case basis.

2.2 Travel by sea

This section was prepared in collaboration with the International Society of Travel Medicine.

The passenger shipping industry (cruise ships and ferries) has expanded considerably in recent decades. In 2008, 13 million passengers worldwide travelled on cruise ships. Cruise itineraries cover all continents, including areas that are not easily accessible by other means of travel. The average duration of a cruise is about 7 days, but cruise voyages can last from several hours to several months. A typical cruise ship now carries up to 3000 passengers and 1000 crew.

The revised International Health Regulations (2005) address health requirements for ship operations. There are global standards regarding ship and port sanitation and disease surveillance, as well as response to infectious diseases. Guidance is given on provision of safe water and food, on vector and rodent control, and on waste disposal. According to Article 8 of the International Labour Organization Convention (No. 164) "Concerning Health Protection and Medical Care for Seafarers" (1987), vessels carrying more than 100 crew members on an international voyage of 3 days or longer must provide a physician for care of the crew. These regulations do not apply to passenger vessels and ferries sailing for less than 3 days, even though the number of crew and passengers may exceed 1000. Ferries often do not have an emergency room but a ship's officer or a nurse is designated to provide medical help. The contents of the ship's medical chest must be in accordance with the international recommendations and national laws for ocean-going trade vessels, but there are no special requirements for additional drugs for passenger ships.

The average traveller on a cruise line is 45–50 years of age. Senior citizens represent about one-third of passengers. Cruises of longer duration often attract older travellers, a group likely to have more chronic medical problems, such as heart and lung disease. More than half of all emergency visits to health clinics on board are made by passengers who are over 65 years of age; the most common health problems are respiratory tract infection, injuries, motion sickness and gastrointestinal illness. Extended periods away from home, especially days at sea, make it essential for passengers to stock up with sufficient medical supplies. Prescription medicines should be carried in the original packages or containers, together with a letter from a medical practitioner attesting to the traveller's need for those medicines. Cruise ship travellers who may require particular medical treatment should consult their health-care providers before booking.

It is important to view a ship's medical facility as an infirmary and not as a hospital. Although most of the medical conditions that arise aboard ship can be treated as they would be at an ambulatory care centre at home, more severe problems may require the patient to be treated in a fully staffed and equipped land-based hospital after stabilization on the ship. Knowledge of the type and quality of medical facilities along the itinerary is important to determine whether passengers or crew members can be sent ashore for additional care or need to be evacuated by air back to the home port. Most cruise vessels do not have assigned space for a dental office, and very few have a resident dentist.

The rapid movement of cruise ships from one port to another, with the likelihood of wide variations in sanitation standards and infectious disease exposure risks, often results in the introduction of communicable diseases by embarking passengers and crew members. In the relatively closed and crowded environment of a ship, disease may spread to other passengers and crew members; diseases may also be disseminated to the home communities of disembarking passengers and crew members. More than 100 disease outbreaks associated with ships have been identified in the past 30 years. This is probably an underestimate because many outbreaks are not reported and some may go undetected. Outbreaks of measles, rubella, varicella, meningococcal meningitis, hepatitis A, legionellosis, and respiratory and gastrointestinal illnesses among ship passengers have been reported. Such outbreaks are of concern because of their potentially serious health consequences and high costs to the industry. In recent years, influenza and norovirus outbreaks have been public health challenges for the cruise industry.

2.2.1 Communicable diseases

Gastrointestinal disease

Most of the detected gastrointestinal disease outbreaks associated with cruise ships have been linked to food or water consumed on board. Factors that have contributed to outbreaks include contaminated bunkered water, inadequate disinfection of water, potable water contaminated by sewage on ship, poor design and construction of storage tanks for potable water, deficiencies in food handling, preparation and cooking, and use of seawater in the galley.

Norovirus is the most common pathogen implicated in outbreaks. Symptoms often start with sudden onset of vomiting and/or diarrhoea. There may be fever, abdominal cramps and malaise. The virus can spread in food or water or from person to person; it is highly infectious and in an outbreak on a cruise ship, more than 80% of the passengers can be affected. To prevent or reduce outbreaks of gastroenteritis caused by norovirus, ships are enhancing food and water sanitation measures and disinfection of surfaces; more ships are providing hand gel dispensers at strategic locations throughout the ship and passengers and crew are urged to use them. Some cruise companies ask that those who present with gastrointestinal symptoms at on-board medical centres be put into isolation until at least 24 h after their last symptoms, and some ships also isolate asymptomatic contacts for 24 h.

Influenza and other respiratory tract infections

Respiratory tract infections are frequent among cruise ship passengers. Travellers from areas of the world where influenza viruses are in seasonal circulation may introduce such viruses to regions of the world where influenza is not in seasonal circulation. Crew members who serve passengers may become reservoirs for influenza infection and may transmit disease to passengers on subsequent cruises.

Legionellosis

Legionellosis (Legionnaires' disease) is a potentially fatal form of pneumonia, first recognized in 1976. The disease is normally contracted by inhaling *Legionella* bacteria deep into the lungs. *Legionella* species can be found in tiny droplets of water (aerosols) or in droplet nuclei (the particles left after water has evaporated). More than 50 incidents of legionellosis, involving over 200 cases, have been associated with ships during the past three decades. For example, an outbreak of legionellosis occurring on a cruise ship in 1994, resulted in 50 passengers on nine other cruises becoming infected, with one death. The disease was linked to a whirlpool spa on the ship. Other sources have been potable water supplies and exposure during port layovers.

Prevention and control depend on proper disinfection, filtration and storage of source water, and on designing piping systems without dead ends. Regular cleaning and disinfection of spas are required to reduce the risk of legionellosis on ships.

Other communicable diseases
The outbreaks of varicella and rubella that have occurred underscore the need for travellers to make sure that they are up to date with routine vaccinations; major cruise ship companies are requesting that their crews be vaccinated against varicella and rubella.

2.2.2 Noncommunicable diseases

Because of temperature and weather variations, changes in diet and physical activities, cruise ship passengers – particularly the elderly – may experience worsening of existing chronic health conditions. Cardiovascular events are the most common cause of mortality on cruise ships. Motion sickness can occur, especially on smaller vessels. Injuries and dental emergencies are also frequently reported.

2.2.3 Precautions

The risk of communicable and noncommunicable diseases among cruise ship passengers and crew members is difficult to quantify because of the broad spectrum of cruise ship experiences, the variety of destinations and the limited available data. In general, cruise ship travellers should:

- Before embarking, consult their health care provider, a physician or travel health specialist on prevention guidelines and immunizations, specifically taking into account:
  - the health status of the individual, the duration of travel, the countries to be visited and likely activities ashore;
  - all routinely recommended medical condition age-specific immunizations;
  - influenza vaccination as available regardless of season, particularly if the traveller belongs to one of the groups for whom annual vaccination against influenza is routinely recommended (Chapter 6); the need to provide a prescription for anti-influenza medication, for treatment or prophylaxis, can then be discussed;

- immunization and other (e.g. malaria) recommendations that apply to each country on the itinerary;
- medication against motion sickness, particularly if the individual is prone to motion sickness.

- See a dentist to make sure they have good oral health and no active problems.

- Consider purchasing a special health insurance policy for trip cancellation, additional medical coverage and/or medical evacuation if necessary.

- Abstain from embarking on a cruise if symptomatic with acute illness.

- Carry all prescription medicines in the original packet or container, together with a doctor's letter (Chapter 1).

- Carry out frequent hand-washing, either with soap and water or using an alcohol-based hand sanitizer.

- Avoid self-medication in the case of diarrhoea or high fever while on board, but report immediately to the ship's medical service.

Further reading

Travel by air

General information related to air travel may be found on the web site of the International Civil Aviation Organization (http://www.icao.int).

Medical Guidelines Task Force. *Medical guidelines for airline travel*, 2nd ed. Alexandria, VA, Aerospace Medical Association, 2003 (available at http://www.asma.org/pdf/publications/medguid.pdf).

Mendis S, Yach D, Alwan Al. Air travel and venous thromboembolism. *Bulletin of the World Health Organization*, 2002, 80(5):403–406.

Summary of SARS and air travel. Geneva, World Health Organization, 23 May 2003 (available at http://www.who.int/csr/sars/travel/airtravel/en/).

The impact of flying on passenger health: a guide for healthcare professionals, London, British Medical Association, Board of Science and Education, 2004 (available at http://www.bma.org.uk/health_promotion_ethics/transport/Flying.jsp).

Tourism highlights: 2006 edition. Madrid, World Tourism Organization, 2006 (available at http://www.unwto.org/facts/menu.html).

Tuberculosis and air travel: guidelines for prevention and control, 3rd ed. Geneva, World Health Organization, 2008 (WHO/HTM/TB/2008.399) (available at http://www.who.int/tb/publications/2008/WHO_HTM_TB_2008.399_eng.pdf).

WHO Research into global hazards of travel (WRIGHT) project: final report of phase I. Geneva, World Health Organization, 2007 (available at http://www.who.int/cardiovascular_diseases/wright_project/phase1_report/en/index.html).

Travel by sea

General information related to travel by sea may be found at the following web sites:

American College of Emergency Physicians: http://www.acep.org/ACEPmembership.aspx?id=24928

International Council of Cruise Lines: http://www.cruising.org/index2.cfm

International Maritime Health Association: http://www.imha.net

Miller JM et al. Cruise ships: high-risk passengers and the global spread of new influenza viruses. *Clinical Infectious Diseases*, 2000, 31:433–438.

Nikolic N et al. Acute gastroenteritis at sea and outbreaks associated with cruises. In: Ericsson CD, DuPont HL, Steffen R, eds. *Traveller's diarrhea*. Hamilton, BC Decker Inc., 2008:136–143.

Sherman CR. Motion sickness: review of causes and preventive strategies. *Journal of Travel Medicine*, 2002, 9:251–256.

Ship sanitation and health. Geneva, World Health organization, February 2002 (available at: http://www.who.int/mediacentre/factsheets/fs269/en/).

Smith A. Cruise ship medicine. In: Dawood R, ed. *Travellers' health*. Oxford, Oxford University Press, 2002:277–289.

WHO International medical guide for ships: including the ship's medicine chest, 3rd ed. Geneva, World Health Organization, 2007.

CHAPTER 3

Environmental health risks

Travellers often experience abrupt and dramatic changes in environmental conditions, which may have detrimental effects on health and well-being. Travel may involve major changes in altitude, temperature and humidity, and exposure to microbes, animals and insects. The negative impact of sudden changes in the environment can be minimized by taking simple precautions.

3.1 Altitude

Barometric pressure falls with increasing altitude, diminishing the partial pressure of oxygen and causing hypoxia. The partial pressure of oxygen at 2500 m, the altitude of Vail, Colorado, for example, is 26% lower than at sea level; in La Paz, Plurinational State of Bolivia (4000 m), it is 41% lower. This places a substantial stress on the body, which requires at least a few days to acclimatize; the extent of acclimatization may be limited by certain medical conditions, especially lung disease. An increase in alveolar oxygen through increased ventilation is the key to acclimatization; this process starts at 1500 m. Despite successful acclimatization, aerobic exercise performance remains impaired and travellers may still experience problems with sleep.

High-altitude illness (HAI) results when hypoxic stress outstrips acclimatization. HAI can occur at any altitude above 2100 m but is particularly common above 2750 m. In Colorado ski resorts, incidence of HAI varies from 15% to 40%, depending on sleeping altitude. Susceptibility is primarily genetic, but fast rates of ascent and higher sleeping altitudes are important precipitating factors. Age, sex and physical fitness have little influence.

The spectrum of HAI includes common acute mountain sickness (AMS), occasional high-altitude pulmonary oedema and, rarely, high altitude cerebral oedema. The latter two conditions, although uncommon, are potentially fatal. AMS may occur after 1–12 h at high altitude. Headache is followed by anorexia, nausea, insomnia, fatigue and lassitude. Symptoms usually resolve spontaneously in 24–48 h and are ameliorated by oxygen or analgesics and antiemetics. Acetazolamide, 5 mg/kg per day in divided doses, is an effective chemoprophylaxis for all HAI; it is started one day before travel to altitude and continued for the first 2 days at altitude. Acetazolamide should not be given to individuals with history of anaphylaxis to sulfonamide drugs.

Only a few conditions are contraindications for travel to altitude; they include unstable angina, pulmonary hypertension, severe chronic obstructive pulmonary disease (COPD) and sickle-cell anaemia. Patients with stable coronary disease, hypertension, diabetes, asthma or mild COPD and pregnant women generally tolerate altitude well but may require monitoring of their condition. Portable and stationary oxygen supplies are readily available in most high-altitude resorts and – by removing hypoxic stress – remove any potential danger from altitude exposure.

Precautions for travellers unaccustomed to high altitudes

- Avoid one-day travel to sleeping altitudes over 2750 m if possible. Break the journey for at least one night at 2000–2500 m to help prevent AMS.

- Avoid overexertion and alcohol for the first 24 h at altitude; drink extra water.

- If direct travel to sleeping altitude over 2750 m is unavoidable, consider prophylaxis with acetazolamide. Acetazolamide is also effective if started early in the course of AMS.

- Travellers planning to climb or trek at high altitude will require a period of gradual acclimatization.

- Travellers with pre-existing cardiovascular or pulmonary disease should seek medical advice before travelling to high altitudes.

- Travellers with the following symptoms should seek medical attention when experiencing, at altitude:
  - symptoms of AMS that are severe or last longer than 2 days;
  - progressive shortness of breath with cough and fatigue;
  - ataxia or altered mental status.

3.2 Heat and humidity

Sudden changes in temperature and humidity may have adverse effects on health. Exposure to high temperature results in loss of water and electrolytes (salts) and may lead to heat exhaustion and heat stroke. In hot dry conditions, dehydration is particularly likely to develop unless care is taken to maintain adequate fluid intake.

The addition of a little table salt to food or drink (unless this is contraindicated for the individual) can help to prevent heat exhaustion, particularly during the period of adaptation.

Consumption of salt-containing food and drink helps to replenish the electrolytes in case of heat exhaustion and after excessive sweating. Travellers should drink enough fluid to be able to maintain usual urine production; older travellers should take particular care to consume extra fluids in hot conditions, as the thirst reflex diminishes with age. Care should be taken to ensure that infants and young children drink enough liquid to avoid dehydration.

Irritation of the skin may be experienced in hot conditions (prickly heat). Fungal skin infections such as tinea pedis (athlete's foot) are often aggravated by heat and humidity. A daily shower, wearing loose cotton clothing and applying talcum powder to sensitive skin areas help to reduce the development or spread of these infections.

Exposure to hot, dry, dusty air may lead to irritation and infection of the eyes and respiratory tract. Avoid contact lenses in order to reduce the risk of eye problems.

3.3 Ultraviolet radiation from the sun

The ultraviolet (UV) radiation from the sun includes UVA (wavelength 315–400 nm) and UVB (280–315 nm) radiation, both of which are damaging to human skin and eyes. The intensity of UV radiation is indicated by the Global Solar UV Index, which is a measure of skin-damaging radiation. The Index describes the level of solar UV radiation at the Earth's surface. The values of the Index range from zero upwards, the higher the Index value, the greater the potential for damage to the skin and eyes and the less time it takes for harm to occur. Index values are grouped into exposure categories, with values greater than 10 being "extreme". In general, the closer to the equator the higher is the Index. UVB radiation is particularly intense in summer and in the 4-h period around solar noon. UV radiation penetrates clear water to a depth of 1 m or more. UV radiation increases approximately 5% for every 300 m altitude gain.

The adverse effects of UV radiation from the sun are the following:

- Exposure to UV radiation, particularly UVB, can produce severe debilitating sunburn, particularly in light-skinned people.
- Exposure of the eyes may result in acute keratitis ("snow blindness"), and long-term damage leads to the development of cataracts.

- Exposure to sunlight may result in solar urticaria – a form of hives associated with itching and redness on areas of skin exposed to sunlight. It can occur within minutes of exposure to the sun and is usually short-lasting.

- Long-term adverse effects on the skin include:
  - the development of skin cancers (carcinomas and malignant melanoma), due mainly to UVB radiation;
  - accelerated ageing of the skin, due mainly to UVA radiation, which penetrates more deeply into the skin than UVB.

- Adverse reactions of the skin result from interaction with a wide range of medicinal drugs that may cause photosensitization and result in phototoxic or photoallergic dermatitis. Various types of therapeutic drugs such as anti-microbials as well as oral contraceptives and some prophylactic antimalarial drugs may cause adverse dermatological reactions on exposure to sunlight. Phototoxic contact reactions are caused by topical application of products, including perfumes, containing oil of bergamot or other citrus oils.

- Exposure may suppress the immune system, increasing the risk of infectious disease, and limiting the efficacy of vaccinations.

Precautions

- Avoid exposure to the sun in the middle of the day, when the UV intensity is greatest.

- Wear clothing that covers arms and legs (covering the skin with clothing is more effective against UV than applying a sunscreen).

- Wear UV-protective sunglasses of wrap-around design plus a wide-brimmed sun hat.

- Apply a broad-spectrum sunscreen of sun protection factor (SPF) 15+ liberally on areas of the body not protected by clothing and reapply frequently.

- Take particular care to ensure that children are well protected.

- Avoid exposure to the sun during pregnancy.

- Take precautions against excessive exposure while on or in water or on snow.

- Check that medication being taken will not affect sensitivity to UV radiation.

- If adverse skin reactions have occurred previously, avoid any exposure to the sun and avoid any products that have previously caused the adverse reactions.

3.4 Foodborne and waterborne health risks

Many important infectious diseases (such as campylobacteriosis, cholera, cryptosporidiosis, cyclosporiasis, giardiasis, hepatitis A and E, listeriosis, salmonellosis, shigellosis and typhoid fever) are transmitted by contaminated food and water. Information on these and other specific infectious diseases of interest for travellers is provided in Chapters 5 and 6.

3.5 Travellers' diarrhoea

Travellers' diarrhoea is a clinical syndrome associated with contaminated food or water that occurs during or shortly after travel. It is the most common health problem encountered by travellers and, depending on length of stay, may affect up to 80% of travellers to high-risk destinations. Travellers' diarrhoea most commonly affects individuals travelling from an area of more highly developed standards of hygiene and sanitation to a less developed one. Diarrhoea may be accompanied by nausea, vomiting, abdominal cramps and fever. Various bacteria, viruses and parasites are the known causes of travellers' diarrhoea, but bacteria are responsible for the majority of cases.

The safety of food, drink and drinking-water depends mainly on the standards of hygiene applied locally in their growing, preparation and handling. In countries with low standards of hygiene and sanitation and poor infrastructure for controlling the safety of food, drink and drinking-water, there is a high risk of contracting travellers' diarrhoea. To minimize any risk of contracting foodborne or waterborne infections in such countries, travellers should take precautions with all food and drink, including that served in good-quality hotels and restaurants. While the risks are greater in poor countries, locations with poor hygiene may be present in any country. Another potential source of waterborne infection is contaminated recreational water (see next section).

It is particularly important that people in more vulnerable groups, i.e. infants and children, the elderly, pregnant women and people with impaired immune systems, take stringent precautions to avoid contaminated food and drink and unsafe recreational waters.

Treatment of diarrhoea

Most diarrhoeal episodes are self-limiting, with recovery in a few days.

It is important, especially for children, to avoid becoming dehydrated. When diarrhoea starts, fluid intake should be maintained with safe liquids (e.g. bottled, boiled or otherwise disinfected water). Breastfeeding should not be interrupted. If moderate to heavy diarrhoeal losses continue, oral rehydration salt (ORS) solution should be considered, in particular for children and elderly individuals.

Amounts of ORS solution to drink

Children under 2 years	$^1/_4$–$^1/_2$ cup (50–100 ml) after each loose stool up to approximately 0.5 litre a day.
Children 2–9 years	$^1/_2$–1 cup (100–200 ml) after each loose stool up to approximately 1 litre a day.
Patients of 10 years or older	As much as wanted, up to approximately 2 litres a day.

If ORS solution is not available, a substitute containing 6 level teaspoons of sugar plus 1 level teaspoon of salt in 1 litre of safe drinking-water may be used, in the same amounts as for ORS. (A level teaspoon contains a volume of 5 ml.)

Antibiotics such as fluoroquinolones (e.g. ciprofloxacin or levofloxacin) may be used as empirical therapy in most parts of the world and usually limit the duration of illness to an average of about one day. However, increasing resistance to fluoroquinolones, especially among *Campylobacter* isolates, may lower their efficacy in some parts of the world, particularly in Asia. In such cases, azithromycin may be taken as an alternative treatment. Azithromycin is a first-line antibiotic therapy for children and pregnant women. When travellers need immediate control of symptoms, antidiarrhoeal drugs such as loperamide may be additionally used, but such antimotility drugs are contraindicated in children aged less than 3 years and not recommended for children under the age of 12.

Prophylactic use of antibiotics is controversial. There is a role for their use in travellers with increased susceptibility to infection, e.g. people with hypochlorhydria or small intestinal pathology and individuals on critical missions. Antidiarrhoeal medicines such as loperamide are always contraindicated for prophylactic use.

Medical help should be sought if diarrhoea results in severe dehydration or has not responded to empirical therapy within 3 days and particularly when bowel movements are very frequent and watery, or when there is blood in the stools, repeated vomiting or fever.

In the event of distressing symptoms suggesting a diagnosis other than travellers' diarrhoea, medical advice should be sought rapidly.

3.6 Recreational waters

The use of coastal waters and freshwater lakes and rivers for recreational purposes has a beneficial effect on health through exercise, and rest and relaxation. However, various hazards to health may also be associated with recreational waters. The main risks are the following:

- Drowning and injury (Chapter 4).

- Physiological:
  - chilling, leading to coma and death;
  - thermal shock, leading to cramps and cardiac arrest;
  - acute exposure to heat and UV radiation in sunlight: heat exhaustion, sunburn, sunstroke;
  - cumulative exposure to sun (skin cancers, cataract).

- Infection:
  - ingestion or inhalation of, or contact with, pathogenic bacteria, fungi, parasites and viruses;
  - bites by mosquitoes and other insect vectors of infectious diseases.

- Poisoning and toxicoses:
  - ingestion or inhalation of, or contact with, chemically contaminated water, including oil slicks;
  - stings or bites of venomous animals;
  - ingestion or inhalation of, or contact with, blooms of toxigenic plankton.

3.6.1 Exposure to cold: immersion hypothermia

Cold, rather than simple drowning, is the main cause of death following immersion. When the body temperature falls (hypothermia), there is confusion followed by loss of consciousness, so that the head goes under water leading to drowning. With a life jacket capable of keeping the individual's head out of water, drowning is avoided, but death due directly to hypothermic cardiac arrest will soon follow. However, wearing warm clothing as well as a life jacket can greatly prolong survival in cold water. Children, particularly boys, have less fat than adults and chill very rapidly in cool or cold water.

Swimming is difficult in very cold water (5 °C or below), and even good swimmers can drown suddenly if they attempt to swim even short distances in water at these temperatures without a life jacket. Life jackets or some other form of flotation aid should always be worn in small craft, particularly by children and young men.

Alcohol, even in small amounts, can cause hypoglycaemia if consumed without food and after exercise. It causes confusion and disorientation and also, in cold surroundings, a rapid fall in body temperature. Unless sufficient food is eaten at the same time, small amounts of alcohol can be exceedingly dangerous on long-distance swims, as well as after rowing or other strenuous and prolonged water-sports exercise.

Those engaging in winter activities on water, such as skating and fishing, should be aware that whole-body immersion must be avoided. Accidental immersion in water at or close to freezing temperatures is extremely dangerous: the median lethal immersion time (time to death) is less than 30 min for children and most adults.

Immediate treatment is much more important than any later action in reviving victims of immersion hypothermia. A hot bath (the temperature no higher than the immersed hand will tolerate) is the most effective measure. In case of drowning, cardiac arrest and cessation of breathing should be treated by giving immediate external cardiac massage and artificial ventilation. Cardiac massage should not be applied unless the heart has stopped. People who have inhaled water should always be sent to hospital to check for pulmonary complications.

3.6.2 Infection

In coastal waters, infection may result from ingestion or inhalation of, or contact with, pathogenic microorganisms, which may be naturally present, carried by people or animals using the water, or present as a result of faecal contamination. The most common consequences among travellers are diarrhoeal disease, acute febrile respiratory disease and ear infections. Skin abrasions from corals are frequently contaminated by live coral organisms and severe skin infections can ensue quickly.

In fresh waters, leptospirosis may be spread by the urine of infected rodents, causing human infection through contact with broken skin or mucous membranes. In areas endemic for schistosomiasis, infection may be acquired by penetration of the skin by larvae during swimming or wading (Chapter 5).

In swimming pools and spas, infection may occur if treatment and disinfection of the water are inadequate. Diarrhoea, gastroenteritis and throat infections may result from contact with contaminated water. Appropriate use of chlorine and other disinfectants controls most viruses and bacteria in water. However, the parasites *Giardia* and *Cryptosporidium*, which are shed in large numbers by infected individuals, are highly resistant to routine disinfection procedures; they are inactivated by ozone or eliminated by filtration.

Contamination of spas and whirlpools may lead to infection by *Legionella* and *Pseudomonas aeruginosa*. Otitis externa and infections of the urinary tract, respiratory tract, wounds and cornea have also been linked to spas.

Direct person-to-person contact or physical contact with contaminated surfaces in the vicinity of pools and spas may spread the viruses that cause molluscum contagiosum and cutaneous papillomas (warts); fungal infections of the hair, fingernails and skin, notably tinea pedis (athlete's foot), are spread in a similar manner.

3.6.3 Precautions

- Adopt safe behaviour in all recreational waters (Chapter 4).
- Avoid consumption of alcohol before and during any activities in or near recreational waters.
- Provide constant supervision of children in the vicinity of recreational waters.
- Avoid temperature extremes in spas, saunas, etc; this is particularly important for users with pre-existing medical conditions, pregnant women and young children.
- Avoid contact with contaminated waters.
- Apply antiseptic to coral cuts and abrasions.
- Avoid swallowing any water.
- Obtain advice locally about the presence of potentially dangerous aquatic animals.
- Wear shoes when walking on shores, riverbanks and muddy terrain.

3.7 Animals and insects

3.7.1 Mammals

Undomesticated animals tend to avoid contact with humans and most do not attack unless provoked. Some large carnivores, however, are aggressive and may attack. Animals suffering from rabies often become aggressive and may attack without provocation. Wild animals may become aggressive if there is territorial intrusion, particularly when they are protecting their young. Animal bites may cause serious injury and may also result in transmission of disease.

Rabies is the most important infectious health hazard from animal bites. In many developing countries, rabies is transmitted mainly by dogs, but many other species of mammals can be infected by the rabies virus. After any animal bite, the wound should be thoroughly cleansed with disinfectant or with soap or detergent and water, and medical or veterinary advice should be sought about the possibility of rabies in the area. Where a significant risk of rabies exists, the patient should be treated with post-exposure rabies vaccination and immunoglobulin (Chapter 5). A booster dose of tetanus toxoid is also recommended following an animal bite.

Travellers who may be at increased risk of exposure to rabies may be advised to have pre-exposure vaccination before departure (Chapter 6). Pre-exposure rabies vaccination does not eliminate the need for treatment after the bite of a rabid animal, but it reduces the number of vaccine doses required in the post-exposure regimen.

Precautions
- Avoid direct contact with domestic animals in areas where rabies occurs, and with all wild and captive animals.
- Avoid behaviour that may startle, frighten or threaten an animal.
- Ensure that children do not approach, touch or otherwise provoke any animal.
- Treat any animal bite immediately by washing with disinfectant or soap and seek medical advice.
- If a significant risk of exposure to rabies is foreseen, seek medical advice before travelling.

Travellers with accompanying animals should be aware that dogs (and, for some countries, cats) must be vaccinated against rabies in order to be allowed to cross international borders. A number of rabies-free countries have additional requirements. Before taking an animal abroad, the traveller should ascertain the regulatory requirements of the countries of destination and transit.

3.7.2 Snakes, scorpions and spiders

Travellers to tropical, subtropical and desert areas should be aware of the possible presence of venomous snakes, scorpions and spiders. Local advice should be sought about risks in the areas to be visited. Most venomous species are particularly active at night.

Venom from snake and spider bites and from scorpion stings has various effects in addition to tissue damage in the vicinity of the bite. Neurotoxins are present in the venom of both terrestrial and aquatic snakes, and also often in the venom of scorpions and spiders. Neurotoxins cause weakness and paralysis. Venom contacting the eyes causes severe damage and may result in blindness. Most snake venoms affect blood coagulation, which may result in haemorrhage and reduced blood pressure. Toxins in the hair of spiders such as tarantulas may cause intense irritation on contact with the skin.

Poisoning by a venomous snake, scorpion or spider is a medical emergency requiring immediate attention. The patient should be moved to the nearest medical facility as quickly as possible. First-aid measures involve immobilizing the entire affected limb with splints and firm, but not tight, bandaging to limit the spread of toxin in the body and the amount of local tissue damage. However, bandaging is not recommended if local swelling and tissue damage are present in the vicinity of the bite. Other traditional first-aid measures (incisions and suction, tourniquets and compression) are harmful and should not be used.

The decision to use antivenom should be taken only by qualified medical personnel. Antivenom should be administered in a medical facility and should be given only if its stated range of specificity includes the species responsible for the bite.

Precautions
- Obtain local advice about the possible presence of venomous snakes, scorpions and spiders in the area.
- Avoid walking barefoot or in open sandals in terrain where venomous snakes, scorpions or spiders may be present; wear boots or closed shoes and long trousers.
- Avoid placing hands or feet where snakes, spiders or scorpions may be hiding.
- Be particularly careful outdoors at night.
- Examine clothing and shoes before use for hidden snakes, scorpions or spiders. Sleep under a mosquito net.

3.7.3 Aquatic animals
Swimmers and divers may be bitten by certain aquatic animals, including conger and moray eels, piranhas, seals and sharks. They may be stung by venomous cnidaria jellyfish, fire corals, sea anemones, stingrays, weever fish, scorpionfish,

stonefish and invertebrate aquatic species. Severe and often fatal injury results from attack by crocodiles, which inhabit rivers and estuaries in many tropical countries, including the tropical north of Australia. Injuries from dangerous aquatic organisms occur as a result of:

- being in contact with a venomous organism while bathing or wading;
- treading on an animal with venomous spines;
- handling venomous organisms during sea-shore exploration;
- invading the territory of large animals when swimming or at the water's edge;
- swimming in waters used as hunting grounds by large predators;
- interfering with, or provoking, dangerous aquatic organisms.

Precautions

- Obtain local advice on the possible presence of dangerous aquatic animals in the area.
- Avoid behaviour that will provoke attack by predatory animals.
- Wear shoes when walking on the shore and at the water's edge.
- Avoid contact with jellyfish (both live jellyfish in water and dead jellyfish on the beach).
- Avoid walking, wading or swimming in crocodile-infested waters at all times of year.
- Seek medical advice after a sting or bite by a venomous animal.

Treatment

Treatment of envenomation by aquatic animals will depend on whether there is a wound or puncture or a localized skin reaction (e.g. rash). Punctures caused by spiny fish require immersion in hot water, extraction of the spines, careful cleaning of the wound and antibiotic therapy (and antivenom in the case of stonefish). If punctures were caused by an octopus or sea urchin the treatment is basically the same but without exposure to heat. In the case of rashes or linear lesions, contact with cnidaria should be suspected; the treatment is based on the use of 5% acetic acid, local decontamination and corticosteroids (antivenom for the box jellyfish *Chironex fleckeri*), with adequate follow-up for possible sequelae.

3.7.4 Insects and other vectors of disease

Vectors play an essential role in the transmission of many infectious diseases. Many vectors are bloodsucking insects, which ingest the disease-producing microorganism during a blood meal from an infected host (human or animal) and later inject it into a new host at the time of another blood meal. Mosquitoes are important insect vectors of disease, and some diseases are transmitted by bloodsucking flies. In addition, ticks and certain aquatic snails are involved in the life cycle and transmission of disease. The principal vectors and the main diseases they transmit are shown in Table 3.1. Information about the diseases and details of specific preventive measures are provided in Chapters 5, 6 and 7.

Water plays a key role in the life-cycle of most vectors. Thus, the transmission of many vector-borne diseases is seasonal as there is a relationship between rainfall and the existence of breeding sites. Temperature is also a critical factor, limiting the distribution of vectors by altitude and latitude.

Travellers are usually at lower risk of exposure to vector-borne diseases in urban centres, especially if they sleep in air-conditioned rooms. They may, however, be exposed to the vectors of dengue which are frequent in urban centres in tropical countries and which bite mostly during the day. Travellers to rural areas or to areas with low standards of hygiene and sanitation are usually at higher risk of exposure to disease vectors, and personal protection is therefore essential. Evening/night-time activities outdoors may increase exposure to malaria vectors.

Protection against vectors
Travellers may protect themselves from mosquitoes and other vectors by the means outlined in the following paragraphs.

Insect repellents are substances applied to exposed skin or to clothing to prevent human/vector contact. The active ingredient in a repellent repels insects but does not kill them. Choose a repellent containing DEET (N,N-diethyl-3-methyl-benzamide), IR3535 (3-[N-acetyl-N-butyl]-aminopropionic acid ethyl ester) or Icaridin (1-piperidinecarboxylic acid, 2-(2-hydroxyethyl)-1-methylpropylester). Insect repellents should be applied to provide protection at times when insects are biting. Care must be taken to avoid contact with mucous membranes; insect repellents should not be sprayed on the face, applied to the eyelids or lips, or applied to sensitive, sunburned or damaged skin or deep skin folds. Always wash the hands after applying the repellent. Repeated applications may be required every 3–4 h, especially in hot and humid climates when sweating may be profuse. When the product is applied to clothes, the repellent effect lasts longer. However, label in-

Table 3.1 **Principal disease vectors and the diseases they transmit**[a]

Vectors	Main diseases transmitted
Aquatic snails	Schistosomiasis (bilharziasis)
Blackflies	River blindness (onchocerciasis)
Fleas	Plague (transmitted by fleas from rats to humans) Rickettsiosis
Mosquitoes	
Aedes	Dengue fever
	Rift Valley fever
	Yellow fever
	Chikungunya
Anopheles	Lymphatic filariasis
	Malaria
Culex	Japanese encephalitis
	Lymphatic filariasis
	West Nile fever
Sandflies	Leishmaniasis
	Sandfly fever (*Phlebotomus* fever)
Ticks	Crimean–Congo haemorrhagic fever
	Lyme disease
	Relapsing fever (borrellosis)
	Rickettsial diseases including spotted fevers and Q fever
	Tick-borne encephalitis
	Tularaemia
Triatomine bugs	Chagas disease (American trypanosomiasis)
Tsetse flies	Sleeping sickness (African trypanosomiasis)

[a] Based on extensive research, there is absolutely no evidence that HIV infection can be transmitted by insects.

structions should be followed to avoid damage to certain fabrics. Repellents should be used in strict accordance with the manufacturers' instructions and the dosage must not be exceeded, especially for young children and pregnant women.

Mosquito nets are excellent means of personal protection while sleeping. Nets can be used either with or without insecticide treatment. However, treated nets are much more effective. Pretreated nets may be commercially available. Nets should be strong and with a mesh size no larger than 1.5 mm. The net should be tucked in under the mattress, ensuring first that it is not torn and that there are no mosquitoes inside. Nets for hammocks are available, as are nets for cots and small beds.

Mosquito coils are the best known example of insecticide vaporizer, usually with a synthetic pyrethroid as the active ingredient. One coil serves a normal bedroom through the night, unless the room is particularly draughty. A more sophisticated version, which requires electricity, is an insecticide mat that is placed on an electrically heated grid, causing the insecticide to vaporize. Battery-operated vaporizers are also available. Such devices can also be used during daytime if necessary.

Aerosol sprays intended to kill flying insects are effective for quick knockdown and killing. Indoor sleeping areas should be sprayed before bedtime. Treating a room with an insecticide spray will help to free it from insects, but the effect may be short-lived. Spraying combined with the use of a coil, a vaporizer or a mosquito net is recommended. Aerosol sprays intended for crawling insects (e.g. cockroaches and ants) should be sprayed on surfaces where these insects walk.

Protective clothing can help at times of the day when vectors are active. The thickness of the material is critical. Insect repellent applied to clothing is effective for longer than it may be on the skin. Extra protection is provided by treating clothing with permethrin or etofenprox, to prevent mosquitoes from biting through clothing. In tick- and flea-infested areas, feet should be protected by appropriate footwear and by tucking long trousers into the socks. Such measures are further enhanced by application of repellents to the clothing.

Travellers camping in tents should use a combination of mosquito coils, repellents and screens. The mesh size of tent screens often exceeds 1.5 mm, so that special mosquito screens have to be deployed.

Screening of windows, doors and eaves reduces exposure to flying insects. Accommodation with these features should be sought where available.

Air-conditioning is a highly effective means of keeping mosquitoes and other insects out of a room as long as the room has no gaps around windows or doors. In air-conditioned hotels, other precautions are not necessary indoors.

Avoid contact with freshwater bodies such as lakes, irrigation ditches and slow-running streams in areas where schistosomiasis occurs.

3.8 Intestinal parasites: risks for travellers

Travellers may be exposed to a number of intestinal parasitic helminth (worm) infections, particularly when visiting tropical and subtropical countries. The risk of acquiring intestinal parasites is associated with low standards of hygiene and sanitation, which permit contamination of soil, water and foodstuffs with human or animal faeces. In general, the clinical effects are likely to become apparent some time after return from travel and the link with the travel destination may not be apparent, which in turn may delay the diagnosis or lead to misdiagnosis. The following are the main intestinal parasitic helminths to which travellers may be exposed.

- **Hookworms.** Human and canine hookworms, particularly *Necator* and *Ancylostoma* species, may be a risk for travellers, notably in places where beaches are polluted by human or canine faeces. Humans become infected by larval forms of the parasite which penetrate the skin. *A. caninum* produces a characteristic skin lesion, cutaneous larva migrans, which is readily treated by anthelminthics such as albendazole or ivermectin.

- **Tapeworms.** The tapeworm *Taenia saginata* is acquired by consumption of raw or undercooked beef from cattle that harbour the larval form of the parasite. *T. solium* is similarly acquired from raw or undercooked pork. Cattle and pigs become infected with the larval stages of tapeworm as a result of access to human faeces, from which they ingest tapeworm eggs, spread by human tapeworm carriers. Humans, who are the usual definitive host of the parasite, may also become an intermediate host by direct ingestion of *T. solium* eggs in food contaminated by human faeces; this is particularly dangerous, since the larval forms of the parasite cause cysticercosis, which may lead to serious disease. Infection with the larval form of the tapeworm *Echinococcus granulosus* causes cystic hydatid disease; dogs are the definitive host of the adult tapeworm and excrete eggs in their faces. Human infection is acquired by ingestion of eggs following close contact with infected dogs or consumption of food or water contaminated by their faeces.

- **Roundworms and whipworms.** The intestinal roundworm (nematode) parasites *Ascaris lumbricoides* and whipworm *Trichuris trichiura* are transmitted in soil. Soil containing the eggs of these parasites may contaminate foods such as fruit and vegetables, leading to infection if the food is consumed without thorough washing; infection may also be transmitted by the hands following handling of soil-contaminated foods, for instance in street markets, or by contaminated water.

3.9 Summary of practical measures for food and water hygiene and for avoidance of insect bites

3.9.1 Common-sense precautions for avoiding unsafe food and drink

- Avoid food that has been kept at room or ambient temperature for several hours, e.g. uncovered buffet food, food from street and beach vendors.

- Avoid uncooked food, apart from fruit and vegetables that can be peeled or shelled, and avoid fruits with damaged skins.

- Avoid ice unless it has been made from safe water.

- Avoid dishes containing raw or undercooked eggs.

- Avoid ice cream from unreliable sources, including street vendors.

- Avoid brushing the teeth with unsafe water.

- In countries where poisonous biotoxins may be present in fish and shellfish, obtain advice locally.

- Boil unpasteurized (raw) milk before consumption.

- Always wash your hands thoroughly with soap and water before preparing or consuming food.

- Boil drinking-water if its safety is doubtful; if boiling is not possible, a certified, well-maintained filter and/or a disinfectant agent can be used.

- Bottled or packaged cold drinks are usually safe provided that they are sealed.

- Beverages and thoroughly cooked food served at a temperature of at least 60 °C are usually safe.

3.9.2 Treating water of questionable quality

- Bringing water to a visible rolling boil for at least one minute is the most effective way to kill disease-causing pathogens.

- Chemical disinfection of clear, non-turbid water is effective for killing bacteria and viruses and some protozoa (but not, for example, *Cryptosporidium*).

- A product combining chlorine disinfection with coagulation/flocculation (i.e. chemical precipitation) will remove significant numbers of protozoa, in addition to killing bacteria and viruses.

- Turbid water should be cleared of suspended solid matter by letting it settle or filtering it before chemical disinfection is attempted.

- Portable point-of-use (POU) devices such as ceramic, membrane and carbon-block filters remove protozoa and some bacteria. Selecting the most appropriate filter pore size is crucial; a size of 1 µm or less for the filter media pore is recommended to ensure removal of *Cryptosporidium* in clear water. Some filtering devices also employ iodine-impregnated resins to increase their efficiency.

- Unless water is boiled, a combination of methods (e.g. filtration followed by chemical disinfection) is recommended, since most POU filtration devices do not remove or kill viruses. Reverse osmosis (very fine pore filtration that holds back dissolved salts in the water) and ultrafiltration devices (fine pore filtration that passes dissolved salts but holds back viruses and other microbes) can theoretically remove all pathogens.

- A carbon filter can improve taste and, in the case of iodine treatment, can remove excess iodine.

3.9.3 Protection against vectors

- Insect repellents, e.g. repellents containing DEET (*N,N*-diethyl- 3-methylbenzamide), IR3535 (3-[*N*-acetyl-*N*-butyl] aminopropionic acid ethyl ester) or icaridin (1-piperidinecarboxylic acid, 2 (2 hydroxyethyl)-1-methylpropyl-ester).

- Mosquito nets.

- Mosquito coils, aerosol sprays.

- Protective clothing.

- Screening.

- Air-conditioning.

Further reading

A guide on safe food for travellers. Geneva, World Health Organization, 2007 (available at: http://www.who.int/foodsafety/publications/consumer/travellers/en/index.html).

Bites and stings due to terrestrial and aquatic animals in Europe. *Weekly Epidemiological Record*, 2001, 76:290–298 (available at: http://www.who.int/wer/pdf/2001/wer7638.pdf).

Foodborne disease: a focus on health education. Geneva, World Health Organization, 2000. (See annex for comprehensive information on 31 foodborne diseases caused by bacteria, viruses and parasites.)

Guidelines for drinking-water quality, incorporating the first and second addenda. Vol. 1: Recommendations, 3rd ed. Geneva, World Health Organization, 2008 (available at: http://www.who.int/water_sanitation_health/dwq/gdwq3rev/en/index.html).

Guidelines for safe recreational water environments. Vol. 1: Coastal and fresh waters. Geneva, World Health Organization, 2003 (available at: http://www.who.int/water_sanitation_health/ bathing/srwe1execsum/en/index3.html).

Addendum to Guidelines for safe recreational water environments, Vol. 1: Coastal and Fresh Waters, Geneva, World Health Organization, 2009 (available at: http://whqlibdoc.who.int/ hq/2010/WHO_HSE_WSH_10.04_eng.pdf).

Guidelines for safe recreational water environments. Vol. 2: Swimming pools and similar environments. Geneva, World Health Organization, 2006 (available at: http://www.who. int/water_sanitation_health/bathing/bathing2/en/).

Hackett PH, Roach RC. High-altitude illness. *New England Journal of Medicine,* 2001, 345: 107–114.

Pesticides and their application for the control of vectors and pests of public health importance. Geneva, World Health Organization, 2006 (WHO/CDS/NTD/WHOPES/ GCDPP/2006.1) (available at: http://whqlibdoc.who.int/hq/2006/WHO_CDS_NTD_ WHOPES_GCDPP_2006.1_eng.pdf).

Preventing travellers' diarrhoea: how to make drinking-water safe. Geneva, World Health Organization, 2005 (WHO/SDE/WSH/05.07 (available at: http://www.who.int/water_sanitation_health/hygiene/envsan/sdwtravel.pdf).

Rozendaal J. *Vector control: methods for use by individuals and communities.* Geneva, World Health Organization, 1997.

Vectors of diseases: hazards and risks for travellers – Part I. *Weekly Epidemiological Record,* 2001, 76:189–194 (available at: http://www.who.int/wer/pdf/2001/wer7625.pdf).

Vectors of diseases: hazards and risks for travellers – Part II. *Weekly Epidemiological Record,* 2001, 76:201–203 (available at: http://www.who.int/wer/pdf/2001/wer7626.pdf).

WHO advice on ultraviolet radiations: http://www.who.int/uv/en

CHAPTER 4

Injuries and violence

Recent data indicate that almost six million people worldwide lose their lives to injuries and violence each year while many more are injured. Travellers may well be exposed to similar risks and are more likely to be killed or injured through violence or unintentional injuries than to be struck down by an exotic infectious disease (see "10 facts on injuries and violence" at http://www.who.int/features/factfiles/injuries/en/). Traffic collisions are the most frequent cause of death among travellers. The risks associated with road traffic collisions and violence are greatest in low- and middle-income countries, where trauma care systems may not be well developed. Injuries also occur in other settings, particularly in recreational waters in association with swimming, diving, sailing and other activities. Travellers can reduce the possibility of incurring these risks through awareness of the dangers and by taking the appropriate precautions.

4.1 Road traffic injuries

Worldwide, an estimated 1.3 million people are killed each year in road traffic collisions and as many as 50 million more are injured. Projections indicate that road traffic fatalities will be the fifth leading cause of death by the year 2030.

In many low- and middle-income countries, traffic laws are inadequately enforced. The traffic mix is often more complex than that in high-income countries and involves two-, three- and four-wheeled vehicles, animal-drawn vehicles and other conveyances, plus pedestrians, all sharing the same road space. The roads may be poorly constructed and maintained, road signs and lighting inadequate and driving habits poor. Travellers, both drivers and pedestrians, should be extremely attentive and careful on the roads.

There are a number of practical precautions that travellers can take to reduce the risk of being involved in, or becoming the victim of, a road traffic collision.

Precautions

- Obtain information on the regulations governing traffic and vehicle maintenance, and on the state of the roads, in the countries to be visited.

- Before renting a car check the state of its tyres, seat belts, spare wheels, lights, brakes, etc.

- Know the informal rules of the road; in some countries, for example, it is customary to sound the horn or flash the headlights before overtaking.

- Be particularly vigilant in a country where the traffic drives on the opposite side of the road to that used in your country of residence.

- Do not drive after drinking alcohol.

- Drive within the speed limit at all times.

- Always wear a seat-belt where these are available.

- Do not drive on unfamiliar and unlit roads.

- Do not use a moped, motorcycle, bicycle or tricycle.

- Beware of wandering animals.

In addition travellers driving cars abroad should make sure they carry their personal drivers licence as well as an international driving permit and that they have full insurance cover for medical treatment of both illness and injuries.

4.2 Injuries in recreational waters

Recreational waters include coastal waters, freshwater lakes and rivers, swimming pools and spas. The hazards associated with recreational waters can be minimized by safe behaviour and simple precautions.

The most important health hazards in recreational waters are drowning and impact injuries, particularly head and spinal injuries. It is estimated that almost 400 000 deaths are caused by drowning every year. In addition, many more cases of "non-fatal drowning" occur, often with lifelong effects on health.

Drowning may occur when an individual is caught in a tide or rip current, is trapped by rising tides, falls overboard from a boat, becomes trapped by submerged obstacles, or falls asleep on an inflatable mattress and is carried out to sea. In swimming pools and spas, drowning or near-drowning and other injuries may occur close to outlets where suction is strong enough to catch body parts or hair so that the head is trapped under water. Drowning in swimming pools may be related to slip–trip–fall incidents leading to loss of consciousness on impact. If the water is not clear it may be difficult to see submerged swimmers or obstacles, increasing the chances of an accident in the water.

Children can drown in a very short time and in a relatively small amount of water. The factor that contributes most frequently to children drowning is lack of adult supervision. Children in or near water should be constantly supervised by adults.

Drowning is also a hazard for those wading and fishing. Falling in cold water, particularly when wearing heavy clothing, may result in drowning as swimming ability is hampered.

Impact injuries are usually the result of diving accidents, particularly diving into shallow water and/or hitting underwater obstructions. Water may appear to be deeper than it is. Impact of the head on a hard surface may cause head and/ or spinal injuries. Spinal injuries may result in various degrees of paraplegia or quadriplegia. Head injuries may also cause concussion and loss of memory and/ or motor skills.

Drowning and impact injuries in adults are frequently associated with alcohol consumption, which impairs judgement and the ability to react effectively.

A detached retina, which can result in blindness or near-blindness, may be caused by jumping into water or jumping onto other people in the water.

Precautions

- Adopt safe behaviour in all recreational waters: use life jackets where appropriate, pay attention to tides and currents, and avoid outlets in spas and swimming pools.

- Ensure constant adult supervision of children in or near recreational waters, including small volumes of water.

- Avoid consumption of alcohol before any activity in or near water.

- Check the depth of the water carefully before diving, and avoid diving or jumping into murky water as submerged swimmers or objects may not be visible.

- Do not jump into water or jump onto others in the water.

4.3 Interpersonal violence

Interpersonal violence is a significant risk in many low-and middle-income countries. Of the approximately 600 000 murders each year, more than 90% occur in low- and middle-income countries. For every murder, scores of people sustain non-fatal injuries requiring medical attention, and hundreds experience more insidious forms of violence and abuse leading to long-term physical and mental health consequences, behavioural disorders and social problems. While there are no epidemiological studies to date that examine how travelling for holiday purposes may increase or reduce involvement in violence, there is emerging evidence to show how it substantially increases known risk factors for violence, including alcohol and illicit drug use among young adults.

Precautions

- Moderate consumption of alcohol and avoid illicit drugs.
- Avoid becoming involved in verbal arguments that could escalate into physical fighting.
- Leave the scene if you feel threatened by the mood and tone set by other people's behaviour.
- Avoid going to someone else's private home or hotel room until you know them well.
- Be alert to the possibility of muggings during the day as well as at night.
- Keep jewellery, cameras and other items of value out of sight and do not carry large sums of money on your person.
- Avoid isolated beaches and other remote areas.
- Use taxis from authorized ranks only.
- Avoid driving at night and never travel alone.
- Keep car doors locked and windows shut.
- Be particularly alert when waiting at traffic lights.
- Park in well-lit areas and do not pick up strangers.
- Employ the services of a local guide/interpreter or local driver when travelling to remote areas.
- Vehicle hijacking is a recognized risk in a number of countries. If stopped by armed robbers, make no attempt to resist and keep hands where the attackers can see them at all times.

Further reading

WHO information on violence and injury prevention available at: http://www.who.int/violence_injury_prevention/en

CHAPTER 5

Infectious diseases of potential risk for travellers

Depending on the travel destination, travellers may be exposed to a number of infectious diseases; exposure depends on the presence of infectious agents in the area to be visited. The risk of becoming infected will vary according to the purpose of the trip and the itinerary within the area, the standards of accommodation, hygiene and sanitation, as well as the behaviour of the traveller. In some instances, disease can be prevented by vaccination, but there are some infectious diseases, including some of the most important and most dangerous, for which no vaccines exist.

General precautions can greatly reduce the risk of exposure to infectious agents and should always be taken for visits to any destination where there is a significant risk of exposure, regardless of whether any vaccinations or medication have been administered.

5.1 Modes of transmission and general precautions

The modes of transmission for different infectious diseases and the corresponding general precautions are outlined in the following paragraphs.

5.1.1 Foodborne and waterborne diseases

Foodborne and waterborne diseases are transmitted by consumption of contaminated food and drink. The risk of infection is reduced by taking hygienic precautions with all food, drink and drinking-water consumed when travelling and by avoiding direct contact with polluted recreational waters (Chapter 3). Examples of diseases acquired through food and water consumption are travellers' diarrhoea, hepatitis A, typhoid fever and cholera.

5.1.2 Vector-borne diseases

A number of particularly serious infections are transmitted by insects such as mosquitoes and other vectors such as ticks. The risk of infection can be reduced by taking precautions to avoid insect bites and contact with other vectors in pla-

55

ces where infection is likely to be present (Chapter 3). Examples of vector-borne diseases are malaria, yellow fever, dengue, Japanese encephalitis, chikungunya and tick-borne encephalitis.

5.1.3 Zoonoses (diseases transmitted by animals)

Zoonoses include many infections that can be transmitted to humans through animal bites or contact with animals, contaminated body fluids or faeces, or by consumption of foods of animal origin, particularly meat and milk products. The risk of infection can be reduced by avoiding close contact with any animals – including wild, captive and domestic animals – in places where infection is likely to be present. Particular care should be taken to prevent children from approaching or touching animals. Examples of zoonoses are rabies, tularaemia, brucellosis, leptospirosis and certain viral haemorrhagic fevers.

5.1.4 Sexually transmitted diseases

Sexually transmitted infections are passed from person to person through unsafe sexual practices. The risk of infection can be reduced by avoiding casual and unprotected sexual intercourse and by use of condoms. Examples of sexually transmitted diseases are hepatitis B, HIV/AIDS and syphilis.

5.1.5 Bloodborne diseases

Bloodborne diseases are transmitted by direct contact with infected blood or other body fluids. The risk of infection can be reduced by avoiding direct contact with blood and body fluids, by avoiding the use of potentially contaminated needles and syringes for injection or any other medical or cosmetic procedure that penetrates the skin (including acupuncture, piercing and tattooing), and by avoiding transfusion of unsafe blood (Chapter 8). Examples of bloodborne diseases are hepatitis B and C, HIV/AIDS and malaria.

5.1.6 Airborne diseases

Airborne transmission occurs when droplet nuclei <5 μm in size are disseminated in the air. These droplet nuclei can remain suspended in the air for some time. Droplet nuclei are the residuals of evaporated droplets. Diseases spread by this mode include open/active pulmonary tuberculosis (TB), measles, varicella (chickenpox), pulmonary plague and haemorrhagic fever with pneumonia.

Droplet transmission occurs when there is adequate contact between the mucous membranes of the nose and mouth or conjunctivae of a susceptible individual and large particle droplets (>5 μm). Droplets are usually generated by the infected individual during coughing, sneezing or talking or when health care workers undertake procedures such as tracheal suctioning. Diseases transmitted by this route include pneumonia, pertussis, diphtheria, SARS, mumps and meningitis.

5.1.7 Diseases transmitted via soil

Soil-transmitted diseases include those caused by dormant forms (spores) of infectious agents, which can cause infection by contact with broken skin (minor cuts, scratches, etc). The risk of infection can be reduced by protecting the skin from direct contact with soil in places where soil transmitted infections are likely to be present. Examples of bacterial diseases transmitted via soil are anthrax and tetanus. Certain intestinal parasitic infections, such as ascariasis and trichuriasis, are transmitted via soil, and infection may result from consumption of soil-contaminated vegetables. Fungal infections may be acquired by inhalation of contaminated soil.

5.2 Specific infectious diseases involving potential health risks for travellers

The main infectious diseases to which travellers may be exposed, and precautions for each, are detailed on the following pages. Information on malaria, one of the most important infectious disease threats for travellers, is provided in Chapter 7. The infectious diseases described in this chapter have been selected on the basis of the following criteria:

— diseases that have a sufficiently high global or regional prevalence to constitute a significant risk for travellers;
— diseases that are severe and life-threatening, even though the risk of exposure may be low for most travellers;
— diseases for which the perceived risk may be much greater than the real risk, and which may therefore cause anxiety to travellers;
— diseases that involve a public health risk due to transmission of infection to others by the infected traveller.

Information about available vaccines and indications for their use by travellers is provided in Chapter 6. Advice concerning the diseases for which vaccination is routinely administered in childhood, i.e. diphtheria, measles, mumps and rubella, pertussis, poliomyelitis and tetanus, and the use of the corresponding vaccines later in life and for travel, is also given in Chapter 6. These diseases are not included in this chapter.

The most common infectious illness to affect travellers, namely travellers' diarrhoea, is covered in Chapter 3. Because travellers' diarrhoea can be caused by many different foodborne and waterborne infectious agents, for which treatment and precautions are essentially the same, the illness is not included with the specific infectious diseases.

Some of the diseases included in this chapter, such as brucellosis, HIV/AIDS, leishmaniasis and TB, have prolonged and variable incubation periods. Clinical manifestations of these diseases may appear long after the return from travel, so that the link with the travel destination where the infection was acquired may not be readily apparent.

The list below does not include vaccine-preventable diseases (Chapter 6).

AMOEBIASIS

Cause	Caused by the protozoan parasite *Entamoeba histolytica*.
Transmission	Transmission occurs via the faecal oral route, either directly by person-to-person contact or indirectly by eating or drinking faecally contaminated food or water.
Nature of disease	The clinical spectrum ranges from asymptomatic infection, diarrhoea and dysentery to fulminant colitis and peritonitis as well as extraintestinal amoebiasis.

Acute amoebiasis can present as diarrhoea or dysentery with frequent, small and often bloody stools. Chronic amoebiasis can present with gastrointestinal symptoms plus fatigue and weight loss, occasional fever. Extraintestinal amoebiasis can occur if the parasite spreads to other organs, most commonly the liver where it causes amoebic liver abscess. Amoebic liver abscess presents with fever and right upper quadrant abdominal pain. |
| Geographical distribution | Occurs worldwide, but is more common in areas or countries with poor sanitation, particularly in the tropics. |
| Precautions | Food and water hygiene (Chapter 3). No vaccine is available. |

ANGIOSTRONGYLIASIS

Cause	Caused by *Angiostrongylus cantonensis*, a nematode parasite.
Transmission	Transmission occurs by ingesting third-stage larvae in raw or undercooked snails or slugs. It can also result from ingestion of raw or undercooked transport hosts such as freshwater shrimp or prawns, crabs and frogs.

Nature of disease	Ingested larvae can migrate to the central nervous system and cause eosinophilic meningitis.
Geographical distribution	Occurs predominantly in Asia and the Pacific, but has also been reported in the Caribbean. Geographical expansion may be facilitated by infected shipborne rats and the diversity of snail species that can serve as intermediate hosts.
Precautions	Food and water hygiene (Chapter 3), in particular avoid eating raw/undercooked snails and slugs, or raw produce such as lettuce. No vaccine is available.

AVIAN INFLUENZA

Cause	Highly pathogenic avian influenza A (H5N1) virus or other non-human influenza subtypes (e.g. H7, H9)
Transmission	Human infections with highly pathogenic avian influenza A(H5N1) virus occur through bird-to-human, possibly environment-to-human, and, very rarely, limited, non-sustained human-to-human transmission. Direct contact with infected poultry, or with surfaces and objects contaminated by their droppings, is the main route of transmission to humans. Exposure risk is considered highest when there is contact with infected avian faecal material in the environment, especially during slaughter, de-feathering, butchering and preparation of poultry for cooking. There is no evidence that properly cooked poultry or poultry products can be a source of infection.
Nature of disease	Patients usually present initially with symptoms of fever and influenza-like illness (malaise, myalgia, cough, sore throat). Diarrhoea and other gastrointestinal symptoms may occur. The disease progresses within days and many patients develop clinically apparent pneumonia with radiographic infiltrates of varying patterns. Sputum production is variable and sometimes bloody. Multi-organ failure, sepsis-like syndromes and, uncommonly, encephalopathy occur. The fatality rate among hospitalized patients with confirmed H5N1 infection has been high (about 60%), most commonly as a result of respiratory failure caused by progressive pneumonia and acute respiratory distress syndrome. Fatal outcome had also been reported for H7N7 infection in human. However, other avian influenza subtypes (e.g. H9N2) appear to cause mild diseases.
Geographical distribution	Extensive outbreaks in poultry have occurred in parts of Africa, Asia, Europe and the Middle East since 1997, but only sporadic human infections have occurred to date. Continued exposure of humans to avian H5N1 viruses increases the likelihood that the virus will acquire the necessary characteristics for efficient and sustained human-to-human transmission through either gradual genetic mutation or reassortment with a human influenza A virus. Between November 2003 and July 2008, nearly 400 human cases of laboratory-confirmed H5N1 infection were reported to WHO from 15 countries in Africa, south-east and central Asia, Europe and the Middle East.
Risk for travellers	H5N1 avian influenza is primarily a disease of birds. The virus does not easily cross the species barrier to infect humans. To date, no traveller is known to have been infected.

Prophylaxis	Neuraminidase inhibitors (oseltamivir, zanamivir) are inhibitory for the virus and have proven efficacy in vitro and in animal studies for prophylaxis and treatment of H5N1 infection. Studies in hospitalized H5N1 patients, although limited, suggest that early treatment with oseltamivir improves survival. Late intervention with oseltamivir is also justified. Neuraminidase inhibitors are recommended for post-exposure prophylaxis in certain exposed individuals. At present WHO does not recommend pre-exposure prophylaxis for travellers but advice may change depending on new findings. Inactivated H5N1 vaccines for human use have been developed and licensed in several countries but are not yet generally available; however, this situation is expected to change. Some countries are stockpiling these vaccines as a part of pandemic preparedness. Although the vaccines are immunogenic, their effectiveness in preventing the H5N1 infection or reducing disease severity is unknown.
Precautions	In affected countries, travellers should avoid contact with high-risk environments such as live animal markets and poultry farms, any free-ranging or caged poultry, or surfaces that might be contaminated by poultry droppings. Travellers in affected countries should avoid contact with dead migratory birds or wild birds showing signs of disease, and should avoid consumption of undercooked eggs, poultry or poultry products. Hand hygiene with frequent washing or use of alcohol rubs is recommended. If exposure to individuals with suspected H5N1 illness or severe, unexplained respiratory illness occurs, travellers should urgently consult health professionals. Travellers should contact their local health providers or national health authorities for supplementary information.

ANTHRAX

Cause	*Bacillus anthracis* bacteria.
Transmission	Anthrax is primarily a disease of animals. Cutaneous infection, the most frequent clinical form of anthrax, occurs through contact with products from infected animals (mainly cattle, goats, sheep), such as leather or woollen goods, or through contact with soil containing anthrax spores.
Nature of the disease	A disease of herbivorous animals that occasionally causes acute infection in humans, usually involving the skin, as a result of contact with contaminated tissues or products from infected animals or with anthrax spores in soil. Untreated infections may spread to regional lymph nodes and to the bloodstream, and may be fatal.
Geographical distribution	Sporadic cases occur in animals worldwide; there are occasional outbreaks in Africa and central Asia.
Risk for travellers	Very low for most travellers.
Prophylaxis	None. (A vaccine is available for people at high risk because of occupational exposure to *B. anthracis*; it is not commercially available in most countries.)
Precautions	Avoid direct contact with soil and with products of animal origin, such as souvenirs made from animal skins.

BRUCELLOSIS

Cause	Several species of *Brucella* bacteria.
Transmission	Brucellosis is primarily a disease of animals. Infection in people is acquired from cattle (*Brucella abortus*), dogs (*B. canis*), pigs (*B. suis*), or sheep and goats (*B. melitensis*), usually by direct contact with infected animals or by consumption of unpasteurized (raw) milk or cheese.
Nature of the disease	A generalized infection with insidious onset, causing continuous or intermittent fever and malaise, which may last for months if not treated adequately. Relapse is not uncommon after treatment.
Geographical distribution	Worldwide, in animals. It is most common in developing countries, South America, central Asia, the Mediterranean and the Middle East.
Risk for travellers	Low for most travellers. Those visiting rural and agricultural areas in countries or areas at risk may be at greater risk. There is also a risk in places where unpasteurized milk products are sold near tourist centres.
Prophylaxis	None.
Precautions	Avoid consumption of unpasteurized milk and milk products and direct contact with animals, particularly cattle, goats and sheep

CHIKUNGUNYA

Cause	Chikungunya virus – an Alphavirus (family Togaviridae).
Transmission	Chikungunya is a viral disease that is spread by mosquitoes. Two important vectors are *Aedes aegypti* and *Aedes albopictus*, which also transmit dengue virus. These species bite during daylight hours with peak activity in the early morning and late afternoon. Both are found biting outdoors but *Aedes aegypti* will also readily bite indoors. There is no direct person-to-person transmission.
Nature of the disease	The name "chikungunya" derives from a Kimakonde word meaning "to become contorted" and describes the stooped appearance of sufferers with joint pain. Chikungunya is an acute febrile illness with sudden onset of fever and joint pains, particularly affecting the hands, wrists, ankles and feet. Most patients recover after a few days but in some cases the joint pains may persist for weeks, months or even longer. Other common signs and symptoms include muscle pain, headache, rash and leukopenia. Occasional cases of gastrointestinal complaints, eye, neurological and heart complications have been reported. Symptoms in infected individuals are often mild and the infection may go unrecognized or be misdiagnosed in areas where dengue occurs.
Geographical distribution	Chikungunya occurs in sub-Saharan Africa, south-east Asia and tropical areas of the Indian subcontinent, as well as islands in the south-western Indian Ocean. (Map)
Risk for travellers	In countries or areas at risk and in areas affected by ongoing epidemics.
Prophylaxis	There are no specific antiviral drugs and no commercial vaccine. Treatment is directed primarily at relieving the symptoms, particularly the joint pain.
Precautions	Travellers should take precautions to avoid mosquito bites during both day and night (Chapter 3).

Chikungunya, countries or areas at risk

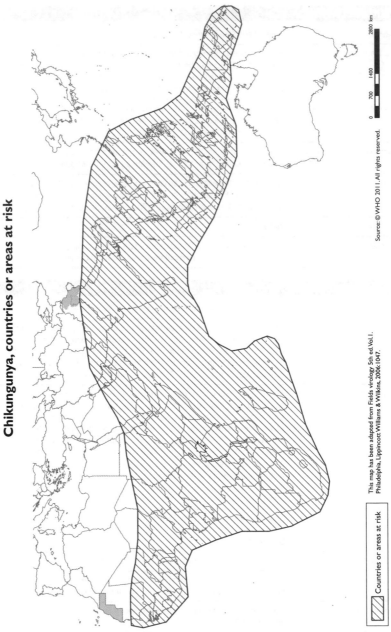

This map has been adapted from Fields virology 5th ed. Vol.1. Philadelphia, Lippincott Williams & Wilkins, 2006:1047.

Countries or areas at risk

COCCIDIOIDOMYCOSIS

Cause	*Coccidioides* spp, a fungus
Transmission	Coccidioidomycosis is transmitted by inhalation of fungal conidia from dust.
Nature of the disease	The spectrum of coccidioidomycosis ranges from asymptomatic to influenza-like illness to pulmonary disease or disseminated disease.
Geographical distribution	Coccidioidomycosis occurs mainly in the Americas.
Risk for travellers	The risk for travellers is generally low. Activities that increase the risk are those that result in exposure to dust (construction, excavation, dirt biking, etc.).
Prophylaxis	No vaccine is available.
Precautions	Protective measures are those that reduce exposure to dust, including wearing well-fitting dust masks.

DENGUE

Cause	The dengue virus – a flavivirus of which there are four serotypes.
Transmission	Dengue is transmitted principally by the *Aedes aegypti* mosquito, which bites during daylight hours. There is no direct person-to-person transmission. Monkeys act as a reservoir host in west Africa and south-east Asia.
Nature of the disease	Dengue occurs in three main clinical forms: ■ Dengue fever is an acute febrile illness with sudden onset of fever, followed by development of generalized symptoms and sometimes a macular skin rash. It is known as "breakbone fever" because of severe muscle, joint and bone pains. Pain behind the eyes (retro-orbital pain) may be present. The fever may be biphasic (i.e. two separate episodes or waves of fever). Most patients recover after a few days. ■ Dengue haemorrhagic fever has an acute onset of fever followed by other symptoms resulting from thrombocytopenia, increased vascular permeability and haemorrhagic manifestations. ■ Dengue shock syndrome supervenes in a small proportion of cases. Severe hypotension develops, requiring urgent medical treatment to correct hypovolaemia. Without appropriate hospital care, 40–50% of cases can be fatal; with timely medical care by experienced physicians and nurses the mortality rate can be decreased to 1% or less.
Geographical distribution	Dengue is widespread in tropical and subtropical regions of central and South America and south and south-east Asia. It also occurs in Africa and Oceania. (Map). The risk is lower at altitudes above 1000 m.
Risk for travellers	In countries or areas at risk and affected by epidemics.
Prophylaxis	There are no specific vaccines or antiviral treatments against dengue fever. Use of paracetamol to bring down the fever is indicated. Aspirin and related non-steroidal anti-inflammatory drugs (NSAIs) such as ibuprofen should be avoided.
Precautions	Travellers should take precautions to avoid mosquito bites both during the day and in the evening in areas where dengue occurs.

Dengue, countries or areas at risk, 2010

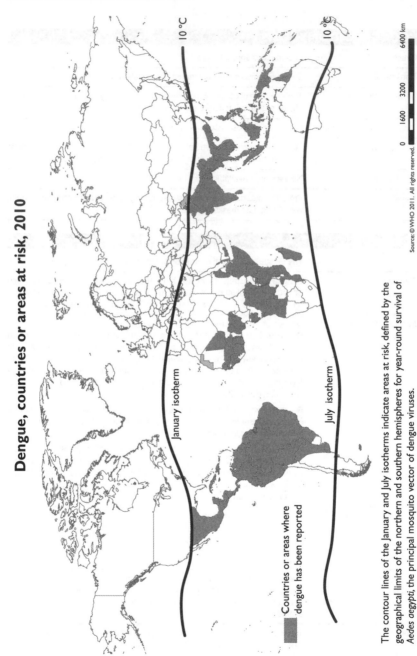

January isotherm

July isotherm

10 °C

10 °C

Countries or areas where dengue has been reported

0   1600   3200   6400 km

The contour lines of the January and July isotherms indicate areas at risk, defined by the geographical limits of the northern and southern hemispheres for year-round survival of *Aedes aegypti*, the principal mosquito vector of dengue viruses.

GIARDIASIS

Cause	The protozoan parasite *Giardia intestinalis*, also known as *G. lamblia* and *G. duodenalis*.
Transmission	Infection usually occurs through ingestion of *G. intestinalis* cysts in water (including both unfiltered drinking-water and recreational waters) or food contaminated by the faeces of infected humans or animals.
Nature of the disease	Many infections are asymptomatic. When symptoms occur, they are mainly intestinal, characterized by chronic diarrhoea (watery initially, then loose greasy stools), abdominal cramps, bloating, fatigue and weight loss.
Geographical distribution	Worldwide.
Risk for travellers	There is a significant risk for travellers in contact with recreational waters used by wildlife, with unfiltered water in swimming pools or with contaminated municipal water supplies.
Prophylaxis	None.
Precautions	Avoid eating uncooked food (especially raw fruit and vegetables) or ingesting any potentially contaminated (i.e. unfiltered) drinking-water or recreational water. Water can be purified by boiling for at least 5 min, or by filtration or chlorination, or by chemical treatment with hypochlorite or iodine (less reliable).

HAEMORRHAGIC FEVERS

Haemorrhagic fevers are viral infections; important examples are Ebola and Marburg haemorrhagic fevers, Crimean–Congo haemorrhagic fever (CCHF), Rift Valley fever (RVF), Lassa fever, Hantavirus diseases, dengue and yellow fever.

Hantavirus diseases, dengue and yellow fever are described separately.

Cause	Viruses belonging to several families. Ebola and Marburg belong to the Filoviridae family; hantaviruses, CCHF and RVF belong to the Bunyaviridae family; Lassa fever belongs to the Arenaviridae family and dengue and yellow fever belong to the Flaviviridae family.
Transmission	Viruses that cause haemorrhagic fevers are transmitted by mosquitoes (dengue, yellow fever, RVF), ticks (CCHF), rodents (Hantavirus, Lassa) or bats (Ebola, Marburg). For Ebola and Marburg viruses, humans have been infected from contact with tissues of diseased non-human primates and other mammals, but most human infections have resulted from direct contact with the body fluids or secretions of infected patients. Humans who develop CCHF usually become infected from a tick bite but can also acquire the virus from direct contact with blood or other infected issues from livestock. RVF can be acquired either by mosquito bite or by direct contact with blood or tissues of infected animals (mainly sheep), including consumption of unpasteurized milk. Lassa fever virus is carried by rodents and transmitted by excreta, either as aerosols or by direct contact. Some viral haemorrhagic fevers have been amplified in hospitals by nosocomial transmission resulting from unsafe procedures, use of contaminated medical devices (including needles and syringes) and unprotected exposure to contaminated body fluids.

Nature of the diseases	The haemorrhagic fevers are severe acute viral infections, usually with sudden onset of fever, malaise, headache and myalgia followed by pharyngitis, vomiting, diarrhoea, skin rash and haemorrhagic manifestations. The outcome is fatal in a high proportion of cases (more than 50%).
Geographical distribution	Diseases in this group occur widely in tropical and subtropical regions. Ebola and Marburg haemorrhagic fevers and Lassa fever occur in parts of sub-Saharan Africa. CCHF occurs in the steppe regions of central Asia and in central Europe, as well as in tropical and southern Africa. RVF occurs in Africa and has recently spread to Saudi Arabia. Other viral haemorrhagic fevers occur in Central and South America. (Maps chikungunya and CCHF)
Risk for travellers	Very low for most travellers. However, travellers visiting rural or forest areas in countries or areas at risk may be exposed to infection.
Prophylaxis	None (except for yellow fever).
Precautions	Avoid exposure to mosquitoes and ticks and contact with rodents or bats. Avoid unpasteurized milk.

HANTAVIRUS DISEASES

Hantavirus diseases are viral infections; important examples are haemorrhagic fever with renal syndrome (HFRS) and hantavirus pulmonary syndrome (HPS).

Cause	Hantaviruses, which belong to the Bunyaviridae family.
Transmission	Hantaviruses are carried by various species of rodents; specific viruses have particular rodent hosts. Infection occurs through direct contact with the faeces, saliva or urine of infected rodents or by inhalation of the virus in rodent excreta.
Nature of the diseases	Hantavirus diseases are acute viral diseases in which the vascular endothelium is damaged, leading to increased vascular permeability, hypotension, haemorrhagic manifestations and shock. Impaired renal function with oliguria is characteristic of HFRS. Respiratory failure caused by acute non-cardiogenic pulmonary oedema occurs in HPS. The outcome is fatal in up to 15% of HFRS cases and up to 50% of HPS cases.
Geographical distribution	Worldwide, in rodents.
Risk for travellers	Very low for most travellers. However, travellers may be at risk in any environment where rodents are present in large numbers and contact may occur.
Prophylaxis	None.
Precautions	Avoid exposure to rodents and their excreta. Adventure travellers, backpackers, campers and travellers with occupational exposure to rodents in countries or areas at risk for hantaviruses should take precautions to exclude rodents from tents or other accommodation and to protect all food from contamination by rodents.

Geographical distribution of Crimean-Congo haemorrhagic fever (CCHF)

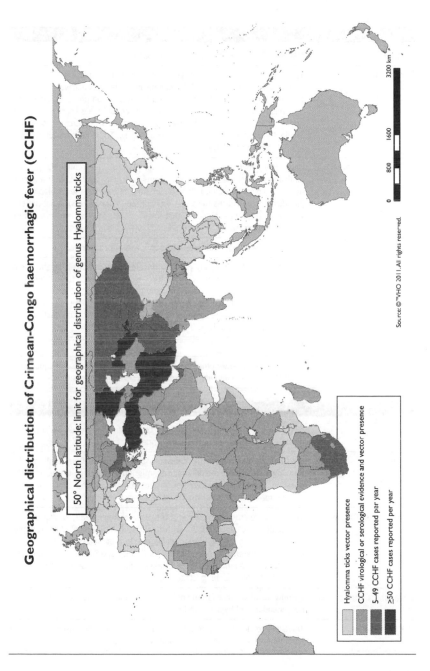

50° North latitude: limit for geographical distribution of genus Hyalomma ticks

Hyalomma ticks vector presence

CCHF virological or serological evidence and vector presence

5–49 CCHF cases reported per year

≥50 CCHF cases reported per year

0   800   1600   3200 km

HEPATITIS C

Cause	Hepatitis C virus (HCV), which is a hepacivirus
Transmission	The virus is acquired through person-to-person transmission by parenteral routes. Before screening for HCV became available, infection was transmitted mainly by transfusion of contaminated blood or blood products. Nowadays transmission frequently occurs through use of contaminated needles, syringes and other instruments used for injections and other skin-piercing procedures. Sexual transmission of hepatitis C occurs rarely. There is no insect vector or animal reservoir for HCV.
Nature of the disease	Most HCV infections are asymptomatic. In cases where infection leads to clinical hepatitis, the onset of symptoms is usually gradual, with anorexia, abdominal discomfort, nausea and vomiting, followed by the development of jaundice in some cases (less commonly than in hepatitis B). Most patients will develop a long-lasting chronic infection, which may lead to cirrhosis and/or liver cancer.
Geographical distribution	Worldwide, with regional differences in levels of prevalence.
Risk for travellers	Travellers are at risk if they practise unsafe behaviour involving the use of contaminated needles or syringes for injection, acupuncture, piercing or tattooing. An accident or medical emergency requiring blood transfusion may result in infection if the blood has not been screened for HCV. Travellers engaged in humanitarian relief activities may be exposed to infected blood or other body fluids in health care settings.
Prophylaxis	None.
Precautions	Avoid the use of any potentially contaminated instruments for injection or other skin-piercing activity and adopt safe sexual practices.

HEPATITIS E

Cause	Hepatitis E virus, which has not yet been definitively classified (formerly classified as a member of the Caliciviridae).
Transmission	Hepatitis E is a waterborne disease usually acquired from contaminated drinking-water. Direct faecal–oral transmission from person to person is also possible. There is no insect vector. Various domestic animals, including pigs, may be reservoirs of hepatitis E.
Nature of the disease	The clinical features and course of the disease are generally similar to those of hepatitis A (Chapter 6). As with hepatitis A, there is no chronic phase. Young adults are most commonly affected. In pregnant women, there is an important difference between hepatitis E and hepatitis A: during the third trimester of pregnancy, hepatitis E takes a much more severe form, with a case–fatality rate reaching 20%.
Geographical distribution	Worldwide. Most cases, both sporadic and epidemic, occur in countries with poor standards of hygiene and sanitation.
Risk for travellers	Travellers to developing countries may be at risk when exposed to poor conditions of sanitation and drinking-water control.

Prophylaxis	None.
Precautions	Travellers should follow the general conditions for avoiding potentially contaminated food and drinking-water (Chapter 3).

HISTOPLASMOSIS

Cause	*Histoplasma capsulatum*, a dimorphic fungus.
Transmission	Via inhalation of spores from soil contaminated with bat guano or bird droppings.
Nature of the disease	Most cases are asymptomatic. Some infections may cause acute pulmonary histoplasmosis, characterized by high fever, headache, non-productive cough, chills, weakness, pleuritic chest pain and fatigue. Most people recover spontaneously, but in some cases dissemination can occur, in particular to the gastrointestinal tract and central nervous system. Risk of dissemination is higher in severely immunocompromised individuals.
Geographical distribution	Worldwide.
Risk for travellers	Generally low except where the traveller may be exposed to bird droppings and bat guano. High-risk activities include spelunking, mining, and construction and excavation work.
Precautions	Avoid bat-inhabited caves. No vaccine available.

HIV/AIDS and other sexually-transmitted infections

Sexually-transmitted infections have been known since ancient times; they remain, worldwide, a major public health problem, compounded by the appearance of HIV/AIDS around 1980. The most important sexually transmitted infections and infectious agents are:

HIV	human immunodeficiency virus (HIV, causing acquired immunodeficiency syndrome (AIDS))
hepatitis B	hepatitis B virus
syphilis	*Treponema pallidum*
gonorrhoea	*Neisseria gonorrhoeae*
chlamydial infections	*Chlamydia trachomatis*
trichomoniasis	*Trichomonas vaginalis*
chancroid	*Haemophilus ducreyi*
genital herpes	herpes simplex virus (human (alpha) herpesvirus 2)
genital warts	human papillomavirus

Travel restrictions

Some countries have adopted entry and visa restrictions for people living with HIV/AIDS. Travellers who are infected with HIV should consult their personal physician for a detailed assessment and advice before travel. WHO has taken the position that there is no public health justification for entry restrictions that discriminate solely on the basis of an individual's HIV status.

Transmission	Sexual infections are transmitted during unprotected sexual intercourse (both heterosexual and homosexual – anal, vaginal or oral). Some of the infectious agents, such as HIV, hepatitis B and syphilis, can also be passed on from an infected mother to her unborn or newborn baby and can be transmitted via

blood transfusions. Hepatitis B and HIV infections may also be transmitted through contaminated blood products, syringes and needles used for injection, and potentially by unsterilized instruments used for acupuncture, piercing and tattooing.

Nature of the diseases	A number of the most common sexually transmitted infections could be included in the following syndromes: genital ulcer, pelvic inflammatory disease, urethral discharge and vaginal discharge. However, many infections are asymptomatic.
	Sexually transmitted infections may cause acute and chronic illness, infertility, long-term disability and death, with severe medical and psychological consequences for millions of men, women and children.
	Apart from being serious diseases in their own right, sexually transmitted infections increase the risk of contracting or transmitting HIV infection. Other viral infections, such as herpes simplex virus type 2 (causing genital ulcer) or human papillomavirus (causing cervical cancer) are becoming more prevalent. The presence of an untreated disease (ulcerative or non-ulcerative) can increase by a factor of up to 10 the risk of becoming infected with HIV. Individuals with HIV infection are also more likely to transmit the infection to their sexual partner if one or both partners already have a sexually transmitted infection. Early diagnosis and treatment of all sexually transmitted infections are therefore important.
Importance and geographical distribution	An estimated 340 million episodes of curable sexually transmitted infections (chlamydial infections, gonorrhoea, syphilis, trichomoniasis) occur throughout the world every year. Regional differences in the prevalence of HIV infection are shown on Map. In high-risk groups, however, such as injecting drug users and sex workers, prevalence rates may be very high in countries where the prevalence in the general population is low.
Risk for travellers	Some travellers may be at an increased risk of infection. Lack of information about risk and preventive measures and the fact that travel and tourism may enhance the probability of having sex with casual partners increase the risk of contracting sexually transmitted infections. In some countries, a large proportion of sexually transmitted infections now occur as a result of unprotected sexual intercourse during international travel.
	There is no risk of acquiring any sexually transmitted infection from casual day-to-day contact at home, at work or socially. People run no risk of infection when sharing any means of communal transport (e.g. aircraft, boat, bus, car, train) with infected individuals. There is no evidence that HIV or other sexually transmitted infections can be acquired from insect bites.
Prophylaxis	Appropriate information about safe sex, risks and preventive measures, and provision of adequate means of prevention, such as condoms, are considered to be the best prevention measures. Vaccination against hepatitis B is to be considered (Chapter 6). Preventive vaccines against oncogenic types of human papillomavirus are now available in some countries. When accidental exposure occurs, post-exposure prophylaxis may be available for hepatitis B and HIV (Chapter 8).
Precautions	The risk of acquiring a sexually transmitted infection can be prevented by abstinence from sex with occasional or casual partners during travel or re-

duced by safer sexual practices such as non-penetrative sex and correct and consistent use of male or female condoms. Condoms also reduce the risk of unwanted pregnancy. Latex rubber condoms are relatively inexpensive, are highly reliable and have virtually no side-effects. Studies on serodiscordant couples (only one of whom is HIV-positive) have shown that, with regular sexual intercourse over a period of two years, partners who consistently use condoms have a near-zero risk of HIV infection.

A man should always use a condom during sexual intercourse, each time, from start to finish, and a woman should make sure that her partner uses one. A woman can also protect herself from sexually transmitted infections by using a female condom – essentially, a vaginal pouch – which is now commercially available in some countries.

To reduce the risk of acquiring hepatitis B and HIV infections, it is essential to avoid injecting drugs for non-medical purposes, and particularly to avoid any type of needle-sharing. Blood transfusions should be given only on the basis of strong (or "clear") medical indications to minimize the risk of transmitting infections such as syphilis, HIV and hepatitis B.

Medical injections, dental care and the use of needles or blades for piercing and tattooing using unsterilized equipment are also possible sources of infection and should be avoided. If an injection is needed, the traveller should try to ensure that single-use needles and syringes come from a sterile package

Patients under medical care who require frequent injections, e.g. diabetics, should carry sufficient sterile needles and syringes for the duration of their trip and a doctor's authorization for their use.

LEGIONELLOSIS

Cause	Various species of *Legionella* bacteria, frequently *Legionella pneumophila*, serogroup I.
Transmission	Infection results from inhalation of contaminated water sprays or mists. The bacteria live in water and colonize hot-water systems at temperatures of 20–50 °C (optimal 35–46 °C). They contaminate air-conditioning cooling towers, hot-water systems, humidifiers, whirlpool spas and other water-containing devices. There is no direct person-to-person transmission.
Nature of the disease	Legionellosis occurs in two distinct clinical forms: ■ Legionnaires' disease is an acute bacterial pneumonia with rapid onset of anorexia, malaise, myalgia, headache and rapidly rising fever, progressing to pneumonia, which may lead to respiratory failure and death. ■ Pontiac fever is an influenza-like illness with spontaneous recovery after 2–5 days. Susceptibility to legionellosis increases with age, especially among smokers and people with pre-existing chronic lung disease and those who are immunocompromised.
Geographical distribution	Worldwide.
Risk for travellers	The risk for travellers is generally low. Outbreaks occasionally occur through dissemination of infection by contaminated water or air-conditioning systems in hotels and other facilities used by visitors.

HIV, estimated prevalence*, 2009

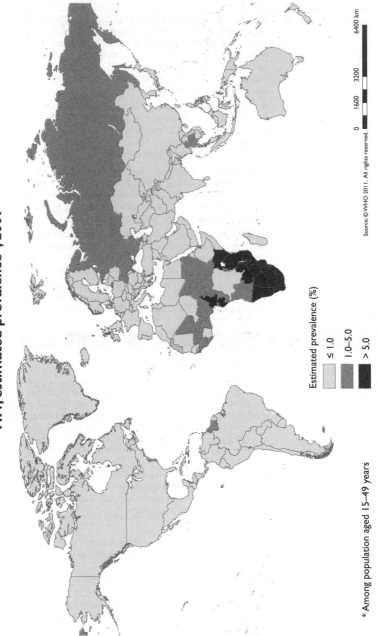

Estimated prevalence (%)

≤ 1.0

1.0–5.0

> 5.0

0   1600   3200   6400 km

* Among population aged 15–49 years

Prophylaxis	None. Prevention of infection depends on regular cleaning and disinfection of possible sources.
Precautions	None.

LEISHMANIASIS (cutaneous, mucosal and visceral forms)

Cause	Several species of the protozoan parasite *Leishmania*.
Transmission	Infection is transmitted by the bite of female phlebotomine sandflies. Dogs, rodents and other mammals, including humans, are reservoir hosts for leishmaniasis. Sandflies acquire the parasites by biting infected reservoirs. Transmission from person to person by injected blood or contaminated syringes and needles is also possible.
Nature of the disease	Leishmaniasis occurs in three main forms:
	■ Cutaneous leishmaniasis. causes skin sores and chronic ulcers. It is generally self-limiting but can be a chronic and progressive disease in a proportion of cases.
	■ Mucosal leishmaniasis: caused by *Leishmania* species in Africa and the Americas, which affect the nasal, oral and pharyngeal mucosa, producing a disabling and mutilating disease.
	■ Visceral leishmaniasis affects the spleen, liver, bone marrow and lymph nodes, producing fever and anaemia. It is usually fatal if untreated.
Geographical distribution:	Many countries in tropical and subtropical regions, including Africa, central and South America, Asia, and the Mediterranean region.
	More than 90% of all cases of cutaneous leishmaniasis occur in Afghanistan, Algeria, Brazil, Colombia, the Islamic Republic of Iran, Peru, Saudi Arabia and the Syrian Arab Republic.
	More than 90% of all cases of mucosal leishmaniasis occur in Plurinational State of Bolivia, Brazil, Ethiopia and Peru.
	More than 90% of all cases of visceral leishmaniasis occur in Bangladesh, Brazil, Ethiopia, India, Nepal and Sudan.
Risk for travellers	Visitors to rural and forested areas in countries or areas at risk.
Prophylaxis	None.
Precautions	Avoid sandfly bites, particularly after sunset, by using insect repellents and insecticide-impregnated bednets. The bite leaves a non-swollen red ring, which can alert the traveller to its origin.

LEPTOSPIROSIS (including Weil disease)

Cause	Various spirochaetes of the genus *Leptospira*.
Transmission	Infection occurs through contact between the skin (particularly skin abrasions) or mucous membranes and water, wet soil or vegetation contaminated by the urine of infected animals, notably rats. Occasionally, infection may result from direct contact with urine or tissues of infected animals or from consumption of food contaminated by the urine of infected rats.

Nature of the disease	Leptospiral infections take many different clinical forms, usually with sudden onset of fever, headache, myalgia, chills, conjunctival suffusion and skin rash. The disease may progress to meningitis, haemolytic anaemia, jaundice, haemorrhagic manifestations and other complications, including hepatorenal failure.
Geographical distribution	Worldwide. Most common in tropical countries.
Risk for travellers	Low for most travellers. There is an occupational risk for farmers engaged in paddy rice and sugar cane production. Visitors to rural areas and in contact with water in canals, lakes and rivers may be exposed to infection. There is increased risk after recent floods. The risk may be greater for those who practise canoeing, kayaking or other activities in water. Outbreaks associated with eco-sports activities have occurred.
Prophylaxis	Doxycycline may be used for prophylaxis if exposure is likely. Vaccine against local strains is available for workers where the disease is an occupational hazard, but it is not commercially available in most countries.
Precautions	Avoid swimming or wading in potentially contaminated waters including canals, ponds, rivers, streams and swamps. Avoid all direct or indirect contact with rodents.

LISTERIOSIS

Cause	The bacterium *Listeria monocytogenes*.
Transmission	Listeriosis affects a variety of animals. Foodborne infection in humans occurs through the consumption of contaminated foods, particularly unpasteurized milk, soft cheeses, vegetables and prepared meat products such as pâté. Unlike most foodborne pathogens, *Listeria* multiplies readily in refrigerated foods that have been contaminated. Transmission is also possible from mother to fetus or from mother to child during birth.
Nature of the disease	Listeriosis causes meningoencephalitis and/or septicaemia in adults and newborn infants. In pregnant women, it causes fever and abortion. Newborn infants, pregnant women, the elderly and immunocompromised individuals are particularly susceptible to listeriosis. In others, the disease may be limited to a mild acute febrile episode. In pregnant women, transmission of infection to the fetus may lead to stillbirth, septicaemia at birth or neonatal meningitis.
Geographical distribution	Worldwide, with sporadic incidence.
Risk for travellers	Generally low. Risk is increased by consumption of unpasteurized milk and milk products and prepared meat products.
Prophylaxis	None.
Precautions	Avoid consumption of unpasteurized milk and milk products. Pregnant women and immunocompromised individuals should take stringent precautions to avoid infection by listeriosis and other foodborne pathogens (Chapter 3).

LYME BORRELIOSIS (LYME DISEASE)

Cause	The spirochaete *Borrelia burgdorferi*, of which there are several different serotypes.
Transmission	Infection occurs through the bite of infected ticks, both adults and nymphs, of the genus Ixodes. Most human infections result from bites by nymphs. Many species of mammals can be infected, and deer act as an important reservoir.
Nature of the disease	The disease usually has its onset in summer. Early skin lesions have an expanding ring form, often with a central clear zone. Fever, chills, myalgia and headache are common. Meningeal involvement may follow. Central nervous system and other complications may occur weeks or months after the onset of illness. Arthritis may develop up to 2 years after onset.
Geographical distribution	There are foci of Lyme borreliosis in forested areas of Asia, north-western, central and eastern Europe, and the USA.
Risk for travellers	Generally low except for visitors to rural areas, particularly campers and hikers, in countries or areas at risk.
Prophylaxis	None.
Precautions	Avoid tick-infested areas and exposure to ticks (Chapter 3). If a bite occurs, remove the tick as soon as possible.

LYMPHATIC FILARIASIS

Cause	The parasitic disease covered is caused by nematodes of the superfamily Filurioidea. Although this group includes lymphatic filariasis (elephantiasis), onchocerciasis (river blindness), loialsis (Calabar swelling) and forms of mansonellosis, the term filariasis is usually used to describe lymphatic filariasis caused by *Wuchereria bancrofti*, *Brugia malayi* or *B. timori*.
Transmission	Lymphatic filariasis is transmitted through the bite of infected mosquitoes, which introduce larval forms of the nematode during a blood meal.
Nature of the disease	Lymphatic filariasis is a chronic parasitic disease in which adult filaria inhabit the lymphatic vessels, discharging microfilaria into the blood stream. Typical manifestations in symptomatic cases include filarial fever, lymphadenitis and retrograde lymphangitis, followed by chronic manifestations such as lymphoedema, hydrocele, chyluria, tropical pulmonary eosinophilic syndrome and, in rare instances, renal damage.
Geographical distribution	Lymphatic filariasis occurs throughout sub-Saharan Africa and in much of south-east Asia, in the Pacific islands and in smaller foci in South America.
Risk for travellers	Generally low, unless travel involves extensive exposure to vectors in countries or areas at risk.
Prophylaxis	None.
Precautions	Avoid exposure to the bites of mosquitoes in countries or areas at risk.

75

MALARIA

Chapter 7.

ONCHOCERCIASIS

Cause	*Onchocerca volvulus* (a nematode)
Transmission	Onchocerciasis (river blindness) is transmitted through the bite of infected blackflies.
Nature of the disease	Onchocerciasis is a chronic parasitic disease, occurring mainly in sub-Saharan western Africa, in which adult worms are found in fibrous nodules under the skin. They discharge microfilaria, which migrate through the skin, causing dermatitis, and reach the eye, causing damage that results in blindness.
Geographical distribution	Onchocerciasis occurs mainly in western and central Africa, also in central and South America.
Risk for travellers	Generally low, unless travel involves extensive exposure to vectors in countries or areas at risk.
Prophylaxis	None.
Precautions	Avoid exposure to the bites of blackflies in countries or areas at risk.

PLAGUE

Cause	The plague bacillus, *Yersinia pestis*.
Transmission	Plague is a zoonotic disease affecting rodents and transmitted by fleas from rodents to other animals and to humans. Direct person-to-person transmission does not occur except in the case of pneumonic plague, when respiratory droplets may transfer the infection from the patient to others in close contact.
Nature of the disease	Plague occurs in three main clinical forms:
	■ Bubonic plague is the form that usually results from the bite of infected fleas. Lymphadenitis develops in the drainage lymph nodes, with the regional lymph nodes most commonly affected. Swelling, pain and suppuration of the lymph nodes produces the characteristic plague buboes.
	■ Septicaemic plague may develop from bubonic plague or occur in the absence of lymphadenitis. Dissemination of the infection in the bloodstream results in meningitis, endotoxic shock and disseminated intravascular coagulation.
	■ Pneumonic plague may result from secondary infection of the lungs following dissemination of plague bacilli from other body sites. It produces severe pneumonia. Direct infection of others may result from transfer of infection by respiratory droplets, causing primary pulmonary plague in the recipients.
	Without prompt and effective treatment, 50–60% of cases of bubonic plague are fatal, while untreated septicaemic and pneumonic plague are invariably fatal.

Geographical distribution	There are natural foci of plague infection in rodents in many parts of the world. Wild rodent plague is present in central, eastern and southern Africa, South America, the western part of North America and in large areas of Asia. In some areas, contact between wild and domestic rats is common, resulting in sporadic cases of human plague and occasional outbreaks.
Risk for travellers	Generally low except in rural areas of countries or areas at risk, particularly if camping or hunting or if there is contact with rodents.
Prophylaxis	A vaccine effective against bubonic plague is available exclusively for individuals with a high occupational exposure to plague; it is not commercially available in most countries.
Precautions	Avoid any contact with live or dead rodents.

SARS (SEVERE ACUTE RESPIRATORY SYNDROME)

Cause	SARS coronavirus (SARS-CoV) – virus identified in 2003. SARS-CoV is thought to be an animal virus from an as-yet-uncertain animal reservoir, perhaps bats, that spread to other animals (civet cats) and first infected humans in the Guangdong province of southern China in 2002.
Transmission	An epidemic of SARS affected 26 countries and resulted in more than 8000 cases in 2003. Since then, a small number of cases have occurred as a result of laboratory accidents or, possibly, through animal-to-human transmission (Guangdong, China).
	Transmission of SARS-CoV is primarily from person-to-person. It appears to have occurred mainly during the second week of illness, which corresponds to the peak of virus excretion in respiratory secretions and stool, and when cases with severe disease start to deteriorate clinically. Most cases of human-to-human transmission occurred in the health care setting, in the absence of adequate infection control precautions. Implementation of appropriate infection control practices brought the global outbreak to an end.
Nature of the disease	Symptoms are influenza-like and include fever, malaise, myalgia, headache, diarrhoea, and shivering (rigors). No individual symptom or cluster of symptoms has proved to be specific for a diagnosis of SARS. Although fever is the most frequently reported symptom, it is sometimes absent on initial measurement, especially in elderly and immunosuppressed patients.
	Cough (initially dry), shortness of breath, and diarrhoea present in the first and/or second week of illness. Severe cases often evolve rapidly, progressing to respiratory distress and requiring intensive care.
Geographical distribution	The distribution is based on the 2002–2003 epidemic. The disease appeared in November 2002 in the Guangdong province of southern China. This area is considered as a potential zone of re-emergence of SARS-CoV.
	Other countries/areas in which chains of human-to-human transmission occurred after early importation of cases were Toronto in Canada, Hong Kong Special Administrative Region of China, Chinese Taipei, Singapore, and Hanoi in Viet Nam.

Risk for travellers	Currently, no areas of the world are reporting transmission of SARS. Since the end of the global epidemic in July 2003, SARS has reappeared four times – three times from laboratory accidents (Singapore and Chinese Taipei), and once in southern China where the source of infection remains undetermined although there is circumstantial evidence of animal-to-human transmission.
	Should SARS re-emerge in epidemic form, WHO will provide guidance on the risk of travel to affected areas. Travellers should stay informed about current travel recommendations. However, even during the height of the 2003 epidemic, the overall risk of SARS-CoV transmission to travellers was low.
Prophylaxis	None. Experimental vaccines are under development.
Precautions	Follow any travel recommendations and health advice issued by WHO.

SCHISTOSOMIASIS (BILHARZIASIS)

Cause	Several species of parasitic blood flukes (trematodes), of which the most important are *Schistosoma mansoni*, *S. japonicum*, *S. mekongi* and *S. haematobium*.
Transmission	Infection occurs in fresh water containing larval forms (cercariae) of schistosomes, which develop in snails. The free-swimming larvae penetrate the skin of individuals swimming or wading in water. Snails become infected as a result of excretion of eggs in human urine or faeces.
Nature of the disease	Chronic conditions can develop when adult flukes live for many years in the veins (mesenteric or vesical) of the host where they produce eggs, which cause damage to the organs in which they are deposited. The symptoms depend on the main target organs affected by the different species, with *S. mansoni*, *S. mekongi* and *S. japonicum* causing hepatic and intestinal signs and *S. haematobium* causing urinary dysfunction. Advanced intestinal schistosomiasis may result in hepatosplenomegaly, liver fibrosis and portal hypertension. Severe disease from uro-genital schistosomiasis may include hydronephrosis and calcification of the bladder. The larvae of some schistosomes of birds and other animals may penetrate human skin and cause a self-limiting dermatitis, "swimmer's itch". These larvae are unable to develop in humans.
Geographical distribution	*S. mansoni* occurs in many countries of sub-Saharan Africa, in the Arabian peninsula, and in Bolivarian Republic of Venezuela, Brazil and Suriname; transmission has also been reported from several Caribbean islands. *S. japonicum* is found in China, in parts of Indonesia and in the Philippines. *S. haematobium* is present in sub-Saharan Africa and in eastern Mediterranean areas. *S. mekongi* is found along the Mekong River in northern Cambodia and in the south of the Lao People's Democratic Republic. (Map)
Risk for travellers	In countries or areas at risk while swimming or wading in fresh water.
Prophylaxis	None.
Precautions	Avoid direct contact (swimming or wading) with potentially contaminated fresh water in countries or areas at risk. In case of accidental exposure, dry the skin vigorously to reduce penetration by cercariae. Avoid drinking, washing or washing clothing in water that may contain cercariae. Water can be treated to remove or inactivate cercariae by paper filtering or use of iodine or chlorine.

Schistosomiasis, countries or areas at risk, 2008

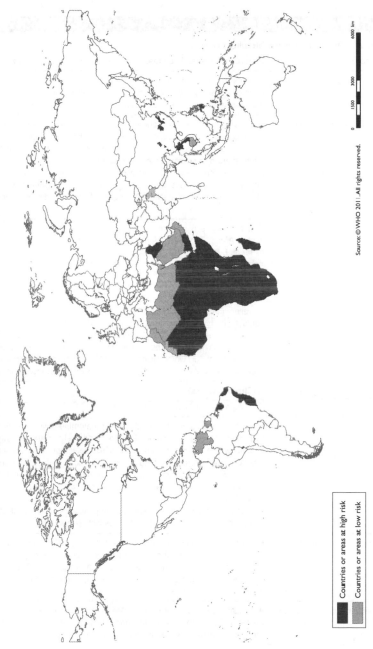

Countries or areas at high risk

Countries or areas at low risk

TRYPANOSOMIASIS

1. African trypanosomiasis (sleeping sickness)

Cause	Protozoan parasites *Trypanosoma brucei gambiense* and *T. b. rhodesiense*.
Transmission	Infection occurs through the bite of infected tsetse flies. Humans are the main reservoir host for *T. b. gambiense*. Domestic cattle and wild animals, including antelopes, are the main animal reservoir of *T. b. rhodesiense*.
Nature of the disease	*T. b. gambiense* causes a chronic illness with onset of symptoms after a prolonged incubation period of weeks or months. *T. b. rhodesiense* causes a more acute illness, with onset a few days or weeks after the infected bite; often, there is a striking inoculation chancre. Initial clinical signs include severe headache, insomnia, enlarged lymph nodes, anaemia and rash. In the late stage of the disease, there is progressive loss of weight and involvement of the central nervous system. Without treatment, the disease is invariably fatal.
Geographical distribution	*T. b. gambiense* is present in foci in the tropical countries of western and central Africa. *T. b. rhodesiense* occurs in eastern Africa, extending south as far as Botswana.
Risk for travellers	In rural areas of countries or areas at risk.
Prophylaxis	None.
Precautions	Travellers in countries or areas at risk should, as far as possible, avoid any contact with tsetse flies. However, bites are difficult to avoid because tsetse flies can bite through clothing. Travellers should be warned that tsetse flies bite during the day and are not repelled by available insect-repellent products. The bite is painful, which helps to identify its origin, and travellers should seek medical attention promptly if symptoms develop subsequently.

2. American trypanosomiasis (Chagas disease)

Cause	Protozoan parasite *Trypanosoma cruzi*.
Transmission	Infection is transmitted by blood-sucking triatomine bugs ("kissing bugs"). Oral transmission by ingestion of unprocessed freshly squeezed sugar cane in areas where the vector is present has also been reported. During feeding, infected bugs excrete trypanosomes, which can then contaminate the conjunctiva, mucous membranes, abrasions and skin wounds including the bite wound. Transmission also occurs by blood transfusion when blood has been obtained from an infected donor. Congenital infection is possible, due to parasites crossing the placenta during pregnancy. *T. cruzi* infects many species of wild and domestic animals as well as humans.
Nature of the disease	In adults, *T. cruzi* causes a chronic illness with progressive myocardial damage leading to cardiac arrhythmias and cardiac dilatation, and gastrointestinal involvement leading to mega-oesophagus and megacolon. *T. cruzi* causes acute illness in children, which is followed by chronic manifestations later in life.
Geographical distribution	American trypanosomiasis occurs in Mexico and in central and South America (as far south as central Argentina and Chile). The vector is found mainly in rural areas where it lives in the walls of poorly-constructed housing.

Risk for travellers	In countries or areas at risk when trekking, camping or using poor-quality accommodation.
Precautions	Avoid exposure to blood-sucking bugs. Residual insecticides can be used to treat housing. Exposure can be reduced by the use of bednets in houses and camps.

TYPHUS FEVER (EPIDEMIC LOUSE-BORNE TYPHUS)

Cause	*Rickettsia prowazekii.*
Transmission	The disease is transmitted by the human body louse, which becomes infected by feeding on the blood of patients with acute typhus fever. Infected lice excrete rickettsia onto the skin while feeding on a second host, who becomes infected by rubbing louse faecal matter or crushed lice into the bite wound. There is no animal reservoir.
Nature of the disease	The onset is variable but often sudden, with headache, chills, high fever, prostration, coughing and severe muscular pain. After 5–6 days, a macular skin eruption (dark spots) develops first on the upper trunk and spreads to the rest of the body but usually not to the face, palms of the hands or soles of the feet. The case fatality rate is up to 40% in the absence of specific treatment. Louse-borne typhus fever is the only rickettsial disease that can cause explosive epidemics.
Geographical distribution	Typhus fever occurs in colder (i.e. mountainous) regions of central and eastern Africa, central and South America, and Asia. In recent years, most outbreaks have taken place in Burundi, Ethiopia and Rwanda. Typhus fever occurs in conditions of overcrowding and poor hygiene, such as in prisons and refugee camps.
Risk for travellers	Very low for most travellers. Humanitarian relief workers may be exposed in refugee camps and other settings characterized by crowding and poor hygiene.
Prophylaxis	None.
Precautions	Cleanliness is important in preventing infestation by body lice. Insecticidal powders are available for body-louse control and treatment of clothing for those at high risk of exposure.

Further reading

Disease outbreak news: http://www.who.int/csr/don/en

Heymann D, ed. *Control of communicable diseases manual*, 18th ed. Washington, DC, American Public Health Association, 2005.

Weekly epidemiological record: http://www.who.int/wer/

WHO information on infectious diseases: http://www.who.int/csr/disease/en

CHAPTER 6

Vaccine-preventable diseases and vaccines

6.1 General considerations

Vaccination is the administration of a vaccine to stimulate a protective immune response that will prevent disease in the vaccinated individual if there is subsequent contact with the corresponding infectious agent. Thus vaccination, if successful, results in immunization: the vaccinated individual has been rendered immune to disease caused by the infectious pathogen. In practice, the terms "vaccination" and "immunization" are often used interchangeably.

6.1.1 Disease prevention

Vaccination is a highly effective method of preventing certain infectious diseases. For the individual, and for society in terms of public health, prevention is better and more cost-effective than cure. Vaccines are generally very safe and serious adverse reactions are uncommon. Routine immunization programmes protect most of the world's children from a number of infectious diseases that previously claimed millions of lives each year. For travellers, vaccination offers the possibility of avoiding a number of dangerous diseases that may be encountered abroad. Immunized travellers will also be less likely to contaminate other travellers or the local population with a number of potentially serious diseases. However, vaccines have not yet been developed against several of the most life-threatening infections, including malaria and HIV/AIDS.

6.1.2 Vaccination and other precautions

Despite their success in preventing disease, vaccines rarely protect 100% of the recipients. The vaccinated traveller should not assume that there is no risk of contracting the disease(s) against which he/she has been vaccinated. All additional precautions against infection (Chapter 3) should be followed carefully, regardless of any vaccines or other medication that have been administered. It is also important to remember that immunization is not a substitute for avoiding potentially contaminated food and water.

6.1.3 Planning before travel

Before departure, travellers should be advised about the risk of disease in the country or countries they plan to visit and the steps to be taken to prevent illness. The risk to a traveller of acquiring a disease depends on the local prevalence of that disease and on several other factors such as: age, immunization status and current state of health, travel itinerary, duration and style of travel. The traveller's individual risk assessment allows a health care professional to determine the need for immunizations and/or preventive medication (prophylaxis) and provide advice on precautions for avoiding disease.

There is no single schedule for the administration of immunizing agents to all travellers. Each schedule must be personalized and tailored to the individual traveller's immunization history, the countries to be visited, the type and duration of travel, and the amount of time available before departure.

Travel is a good opportunity for the health care provider to review the immunization status of infants, children, adolescents and adults. Non-immunized or incompletely immunized travellers should be offered the routine vaccinations recommended in national immunization schedules, in addition to those needed for travel.

Following vaccination, the immune response of the vaccinated individual will be maximal within a period of time that varies with the vaccine, the number of doses required and whether the individual has been vaccinated previously against the same disease. For this reason, travellers are advised to consult a travel medicine practitioner or physician 4–8 weeks before departure in order to allow sufficient time for optimal immunization schedules to be completed. However, even when departure is imminent, there is still time to provide both advice and possibly some immunizations.

6.1.4 Vaccine schedules and administration

The vaccines that may be recommended or considered for travellers are summarized in Table 6.1. Further information on the schedules for administration of these vaccines can be found in the individual vaccines sections, as well as in WHO's position papers on the various vaccines (http://www.who.int/immunization/documents/positionpapers/en/index.html). Summary tables for routine vaccinations can be found at http://www.who.int/immunization/policy/immunization_tables/en/index.html.

Recommendations on time intervals for administration of vaccines requiring more than one dose are provided; some slight variation can be made to accommodate the needs of travellers who may not be able to complete the schedule exactly as recommended. In general, it is acceptable to lengthen the time intervals between doses, but significant shortening of the intervals is not recommended.

6.1.5 Safe injections

The administration of vaccines requires the same high standard of injection safety as any other injection. A sterile needle and syringe should be used for each injection and disposed of safely.

WHO recommends the use of single-use ("auto-disable") syringes or disposable monodose preparations whenever possible. Syringes should not be recapped (to avoid needle-stick injuries) and should be disposed of in a way that is safe for the recipient, the provider and the community.

6.1.6 Multiple vaccines

Inactivated vaccines do not generally interfere with other inactivated or live vaccines and can be given simultaneously with, or at any time in relation to, other vaccines without prejudicing immune responses. Most live vaccines can be given simultaneously provided that they are administered at different anatomical sites. However, if two injected live-virus vaccines are not administered on the same day, the two injections should be separated by an interval of at least 4 weeks. The oral Ty21a typhoid vaccine can be administered simultaneously with, or at any interval before or after, injectable live vaccines.

A number of combination vaccines are now available, providing protection against more than one disease, and new combinations are likely to become available in future years. For routine vaccination of children, the combined diphtheria/tetanus/pertussis (DTP) and measles/mumps/rubella (MMR) vaccines are in widespread use. Other examples of combination vaccines are hepatitis A+B and hepatitis A + typhoid, IPV+DTP, IPV+DTP+Hib, MMR+varicella, IPV+DTP+HepB+Hib.[1] In adults, the combined diphtheria–tetanus vaccine (with reduced diphtheria, Td) is generally used in preference to monovalent tetanus toxoid vaccine. Combination vaccines offer important advantages for travellers by reducing the number of injections required, so aiding compliance. Combination vaccines are just as safe and effective as the individual single-disease vaccines.

---

[1] IPV = inactivated poliomyelitis vaccine; Hib = *Haemophilus influenzae* type b [vaccine]; HepB = hepatitis B [vaccine].

6.1.7 Choice of vaccines for travel

Vaccines for travellers include: (1) those that are used routinely, particularly but not only in children; (2) others that may be advised before travel to countries or areas at risk of these diseases; (3) those that, in some situations, are required by the International Health Regulations.

Most of the vaccines that are routinely administered in childhood require periodic booster doses throughout life to maintain an effective level of immunity. Adults in their country of residence often neglect to keep up the schedule of booster vaccinations, particularly if the risk of infection is low. Some older adults may never

Table 6.1 **Vaccines for travellers**

Category	Vaccine
1. Routine vaccination	Diphtheria, tetanus, and pertussis[c]
	Hepatitis B
	Haemophilus influenzae type b
	Human papillomavirus[a]
	Influenza[b]
	Measles, mumps and rubella
	Pneumococcal disease
	Poliomyelitis
	Rotavirus[a]
	Tuberculosis[e]
	Varicella
2. Selective use for travellers	Cholera
	Hepatitis A[d]
	Japanese encephalitis[d]
	Meningococcal disease[d]
	Rabies
	Tick-borne encephalitis
	Typhoid fever
	Yellow fever[d]
3. Required vaccination	Yellow fever (see Country list)
	Meningococcal disease and polio (required by Saudi Arabia for pilgrims; updates are available on www.who.int/wer)

[a] These vaccines are currently being introduced in some countries.

[b] Routine for certain age groups and risk factors, selective for general travellers.

[c] No longer routine in most industrialized countries.

[d] These vaccines are also included in the routine immunization programme in several countries.

have been vaccinated at all. It is important to realize that diseases such as diphtheria and poliomyelitis, which no longer occur in most industrialized countries, may be present in those visited by travellers. Pre-travel precautions should include booster doses of routine vaccines if the regular schedule has not been followed, or a full course of primary immunization for people who have never been vaccinated.

Other vaccines will be advised on the basis of a travel risk assessment for the individual traveller (Chapter 1). In deciding which vaccines would be appropriate, the following factors are to be considered for each vaccine:

- risk of exposure to the disease
- age, health status, vaccination history
- reactions to previous vaccine doses, allergies
- risk of infecting others
- cost.

Nowadays, only yellow fever vaccination is, in certain situations, required by the International Health Regulations. Yellow fever vaccination is carried out for two different reasons: (1) to protect the individual in areas where there is a risk of yellow fever infection; and (2) to protect vulnerable countries from importation of the yellow fever virus. Travellers should therefore be vaccinated if they visit a country where there is a risk of exposure to yellow fever. They must be vaccinated if they visit a country that requires yellow fever vaccination as a condition of entry; this condition applies to all travellers arriving from (including airport transit) countries or areas at risk of yellow fever.

Vaccination against meningococcal disease is required by Saudi Arabia for pilgrims visiting Mecca and Medina annually (Hajj) or at any time (Umrah).

Some polio-free countries may also require travellers from countries or areas reporting wild polio viruses (updates available at http://www.polioeradication. org/Dataandmonitoring/Poliothisweek.aspx/) to be immunized against polio in order to obtain an entry visa, e.g. Saudi Arabia (Chapter 9). Travellers should be provided with a written record of all vaccines administered (patient-retained record), preferably using the international vaccination certificate (which is required in the case of yellow fever vaccination). The certificate can be ordered from WHO at http://www.who.int/ith/en/.

6.2 Vaccines for routine and selective use

Recommendations on vaccines for routine use are provided by WHO in regularly updated position papers (http://www.who.int/immunization/documents/ positionpapers_intro/en/index.html).

Since the information provided in this chapter is limited, readers are encouraged to refer to these vaccine position papers as well as to national guidelines on routine vaccinations. It is recommended that travellers ensure that all routine vaccinations are up to date. Information on safety of routine vaccines can be found at http://www.who.int/vaccine_safety/en/.

WHO summary tables for recommendations for routine vaccinations can be found at http://www.who.int/immunization/policy/immunization_tables/en/index.html.

Some vaccines need be offered only to travellers who are going to certain specific destinations. The decision to recommend administration of these vaccines will depend on a travel risk assessment for the individual.

CHOLERA	
Cause	*Vibrio cholerae* bacteria of serogroups O1 and O139.
Transmission	Infection occurs through ingestion of food or water contaminated directly or indirectly by faeces or vomitus of infected individuals. Cholera affects only humans; there is no insect vector or animal reservoir host.
Nature of the disease	An acute enteric disease varying in severity. Most infections are asymptomatic (i.e. do not cause any illness). In mild cases, acute watery diarrhoea occurs without other symptoms. In severe cases, there is sudden onset of profuse watery diarrhoea with nausea and vomiting and rapid development of dehydration. In severe untreated cases, death may occur within a few hours due to dehydration leading to circulatory collapse.
Geographical distribution	Cholera occurs mainly in poor countries with inadequate sanitation and lack of clean drinking-water and in war-torn countries where the infrastructure may have broken down. Many developing countries are affected, particularly those in Africa and Asia and, to a lesser extent, those in central and South America (Map).
Risk for travellers	The risk for most travellers is very low, even in countries where cholera epidemics occur, provided that simple precautions are taken to avoid potentially contaminated food and water. Humanitarian relief workers in disaster areas and refugee camps are at risk.
Precautions	Cholera vaccination is not required as a condition of entry to any country. As for other diarrhoeal diseases, all precautions should be taken to avoid consumption of potentially contaminated food, drinks and drinking-water. Oral rehydration salts (ORS) should be carried to combat dehydration in case of severe diarrhoea (Chapter 3).

Vaccine	A vaccine consisting of killed whole-cell *V. cholerae* O1 in combination with a recombinant B-subunit of cholera toxin (WC/rBS) has been marketed since the early 1990s. This killed vaccine is well tolerated and confers high-level (85–90%) protection for 6 months after the second immunization in all vaccinees aged more than 2 years. The level of protection is still about 50%, 3 years after immunization in vaccinees who were aged over 5 years at the time of vaccination. Primary immunization consists of two oral doses 7–14 days apart for adults and children aged 6 years and over. For children aged 2–5 years, three doses are recommended. Intake of food and drinks should be avoided 1 hour before and after vaccination. If the second dose is delayed for more than 6 weeks, vaccination should be restarted. Following primary immunization, protection against cholera may be expected after about 1 week. Booster doses are recommended after 2 years for adults and children aged 6 years and over, and every 6 months for children aged 2–5 years. The vaccine is not licensed for individuals under 2 years of age.
	In studies of travellers to countries or areas reporting cholera outbreaks, WC/rBS was also found to induce approximately 50% short-term protection against diarrhoea caused by enterotoxigenic *Escherichia coli* (ETEC).
	Two closely related bivalent oral cholera vaccines, Shanchol and mORCVAX, are available in India and Viet Nam, respectively. These vaccines are based on *V. cholerae* serogroups O1 and O139 and do not contain the toxin B-subunit. Shanchol and mORCVAX are reported to be safe and efficacious, providing protection against clinically significant cholera in countries or areas reporting outbreaks.

Type of vaccine:	Killed oral whole-cell B-subunit
Number of doses:	Two, at least 1 week (ideally 10–14 days) apart
Contraindications:	Hypersensitivity to previous dose
Adverse reactions:	Mild gastrointestinal disturbances reported
Before departure:	2 weeks
Consider for:	Travellers at high risk (e.g. emergency or relief workers)
Special precautions:	None

DIPHTHERIA/TETANUS/PERTUSSIS

DIPHTHERIA

Cause	Toxigenic *Corynebacterium diphtheriae* and toxigenic *C. ulcerans*.
Transmission	Transmission of bacteria typically residing in the upper respiratory tract is from person to person, through droplets and close physical contact, and is increased in overcrowded and poor socioeconomic conditions. A cutaneous form of diphtheria caused by *Corynebacterium ulcerans* is common in tropical countries and may also be an important source of infection for pharyngeal diphtheria.

Cholera, areas reporting outbreaks, 2009–2010

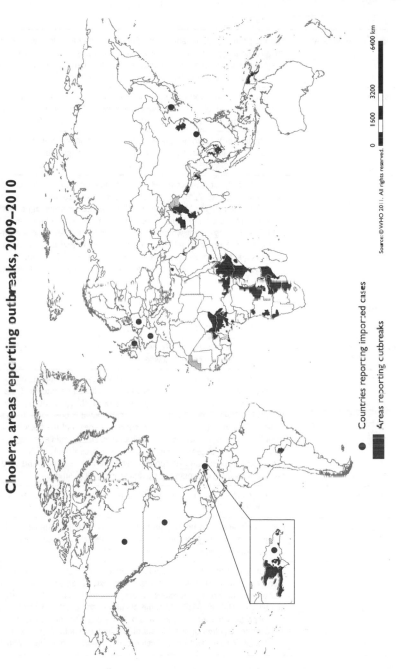

Countries reporting imported cases

Areas reporting outbreaks

0   1500   3200   6400 km

Nature of the disease	The infection commonly affects the throat and may lead to obstruction of the airways and death. There is toxin-induced damage to organs such as the heart. Nasal diphtheria may be mild, and chronic carriage of the organism frequently occurs; asymptomatic infections are common.
Disease burden	Diphtheria is found worldwide, although it is not common in industrialized countries because of long-standing routine use of DTP vaccine. Large epidemics occurred in several east European countries in the 1990s.
Risk for travellers	Potentially life-threatening illness and severe, lifelong complications are possible in non-immunized or incompletely immunized individuals. Diphtheria is more frequent in parts of the world where vaccination levels are low.
Vaccine	All travellers should be vaccinated according to national recommendations. Vaccination against diphtheria is usually given as triple vaccine – DTP or DTaP (diphtheria/tetanus/pertussis or diphtheria/tetanus/acellular pertussis). After the initial course of three doses, additional doses may be given as DT until 7 years of age, after which a vaccine with reduced diphtheria content (Td) is given. Since both tetanus toxoid (see below) and diphtheria toxoid can reasonably be given on a booster basis about every 10 years, there is no reason to use monovalent diphtheria vaccine. In some countries, adult boosters that contain acellular pertussis (TdaP) are being introduced.

TETANUS

Cause	The bacterium *Clostridium tetani*.
Transmission	Tetanus is acquired through exposure to the spores of *Clostridium tetani*, which are present in soil worldwide.
Nature of the disease	The disease is caused by the action of a potent neurotoxin produced by the bacterium (e.g. when present in dirty wounds). Clinical symptoms of tetanus are muscle spasms, initially of the muscles of mastication causing trismus or "lockjaw", which results in a characteristic facial expression – risus sardonicus. Trismus can be followed by sustained spasm of the back muscles (opisthotonus) and by spasms of other muscles. Finally, mild external stimuli may trigger generalized, tetanic seizures, which contribute to the serious complications of tetanus (dysphagia, aspiration pneumonia) and lead to death unless intense supportive treatment is rapidly initiated.
Disease burden	Wounds can become infected with the spores of *Clostridium tetani* anywhere in the world.
Risk for travellers	Every traveller should be fully protected against tetanus. Almost any form of injury, from a simple laceration to a motor-vehicle accident, can expose the individual to the spores.
Vaccine	Tetanus toxoid vaccine is available as single toxoid (TT), combined with diphtheria toxoid (DT) or low-dose diphtheria toxoid (Td), and combined with diphtheria and pertussis vaccines (whole pertussis wP or acellular pertussis aP) (DTwP, DTaP, or TdaP). In some countries, combination vaccines with *Haemophilus influenzae* type b and/or IPV exist. Vaccines containing DT are used for children under 7 years of age and Td-containing vaccines for those aged 7 years and over. Vaccine combinations containing diphtheria

toxoid (D or d) and tetanus toxoid, rather than tetanus toxoid alone, should be used when immunization against tetanus is indicated.

A childhood immunization schedule of 5 doses is recommended. The primary series of 3 doses of DTP (DTwP or DTaP) should be given in infancy, with a booster dose of a tetanus toxoid-containing vaccine ideally at age 4–7 years and another booster in adolescence, e.g. at age 12–15 years. For adult travellers, an extra tetanus toxoid-containing dose will provide additional assurance of long-lasting, possibly lifelong, protection.

All travellers should be up to date with the vaccine before departure. The type of tetanus prophylaxis that is required following injury depends on the nature of the lesion and the history of previous immunizations. However, no booster is needed if the last dose of tetanus vaccine was given less than 5 (for dirty wounds) to 10 years (for clean wounds) previously.

PERTUSSIS

Cause	The bacterium *Bordetella pertussis*.
Transmission	Pertussis (whooping cough) is a highly contagious acute bacterial disease involving the respiratory tract. It is transmitted by direct contact with airborne discharges from the respiratory mucous membranes of infected individuals.
Nature of the disease	Typical manifestations include severe cough of several weeks' duration with a characteristic whoop, often with cyanosis and vomiting. In young infants, the cough may be absent and disease may manifest with spells of apnoea. Although pertussis can occur at any age, most serious cases and fatalities are observed in early infancy and mainly in developing countries. Major complications include pneumonia, encephalitis and malnutrition (due to repeated vomiting). Vaccination is the most rational approach to pertussis control.
Disease burden	WHO estimated that about 16 million cases of pertussis occurred worldwide in 2008, 95% of which were in developing countries, and that some 195 000 patients died from this disease.
Risk for travellers	Unprotected young infants are at highest risk of severe pertussis, but older children, adolescents and adults may also contract the disease (often in mild and atypical form) if they are not fully immunized. Exposure to pertussis is more frequent in developing countries.
Vaccine	All travellers should be up to date with vaccination according to national recommendations. Both whole-cell (wP) and acellular (aP) pertussis vaccines provide excellent protection and are safe apart from minor adverse events. For several decades, wP vaccines have been widely used in national childhood vaccination programmes; aP vaccines, which cause fewer adverse events but are more expensive, are now licensed in many countries. Both wP and aP are usually administered in combination with diphtheria and tetanus toxoids (DTwP or DTaP). Three doses are required for initial protection. Protection declines with time and probably lasts only a few years. A booster dose administered 1–6 years after the primary series (but preferably during the second year of life) is warranted. Some countries now offer an adoles-

cent/adult booster, in particular to health care workers and young parents. Previously unvaccinated adolescents/adults should receive three doses of wP vaccine or aP vaccine with an interval of 2 months between the first dose and the second, and 6–12 months between the second and third doses.

HAEMOPHILUS INFLUENZAE TYPE B

Cause	The bacterium *Haemophilus influenzae* type b (Hib).
Transmission	Respiratory droplets.
Nature of the disease	*Haemophilus influenzae* type b is a common cause of bacterial pneumonia and meningitis and of a number of other serious and potentially life-threatening conditions, including epiglottitis, osteomyelitis, septic arthritis and sepsis in infants and older children.
Disease burden	Hib is estimated to cause at least 8 million cases of serious disease and hundreds of thousands of deaths annually, worldwide. Rarely occurring in infants under 3 months or children after the age of 5 years, the disease burden is highest between 4 and 18 months of age. Hib is the dominant cause of sporadic (non-epidemic) bacterial meningitis in this age group, and is frequently associated with severe neurological sequelae despite prompt and adequate antibiotic treatment. In developing countries, it is estimated that 7–8 million cases of Hib pneumonia occur each year. The disease has practically disappeared in countries where routine vaccination of children is carried out.
Risk for travellers	All unprotected children are at risk, at least up to the age of 5 years.
Vaccine	Vaccination against Hib is recommended for all children over 6 weeks and up to 2 years of age. Infants should receive a primary series of 3 doses, whereas one dose is sufficient in previously unvaccinated children aged 12 months or more. The vaccine is often given as a combined preparation with one or more other vaccines, such as DTP, hepatitis B vaccine or IPV, in routine immunization programmes. Conjugate Hib vaccines have dramatically reduced the incidence of Hib meningitis in infants and of nasopharyngeal colonization by Hib. The vaccine is also available as a single-antigen preparation for use in children who did not receive the vaccine as part of routine immunization. Hib vaccine is not yet used routinely in many developing countries where there is continuing high prevalence of the disease.

HEPATITIS A

Cause	Hepatitis A virus (HAV), a member of the Picornaviridae family.
Transmission	The virus is acquired directly from infected individuals by the faecal–oral route or by close contact, or by consumption of contaminated food or drinking-water. There is no insect vector or animal reservoir (although some non-human primates are sometimes infected).
Nature of the disease	An acute viral hepatitis with abrupt onset of fever, malaise, nausea and abdominal discomfort, followed by the development of jaundice a few days later. Infection in very young children is usually mild or asymptomatic; older

	children are at risk of symptomatic disease. In adults, the disease is often more severe and full recovery may take several months. Case-fatality is greater than 2% for those over 40 years of age and 4% for those over 60.
Geographical distribution	Worldwide, but most common where sanitary conditions are poor and the safety of drinking-water is not well controlled (Map).
Risk for travellers	Non-immune travellers to developing countries are at significant risk of infection. The risk is particularly high for travellers exposed to poor hygiene, sanitation and drinking-water control.
Precautions	Travellers who are non-immune to hepatitis A (i.e. have never had the disease and have not been vaccinated) should take particular care to avoid potentially contaminated food and water.
Vaccine	Hepatitis A vaccination should be considered for all travellers to countries or areas with moderate to high risk of infection. Those at high risk of acquiring the disease should be strongly encouraged to be vaccinated regardless of where they travel.

Current hepatitis A vaccines, all of which are based on inactivated (killed) virus, are safe and highly effective. Anti-HAV antibodies are detectable by 2 weeks after administration of the first dose of vaccine. The second dose – given at least 6 months, and usually 6–24 months, after the first dose – is necessary to promote long-term protection. Results from mathematical models indicate that, after completion of the primary series, anti-HAV antibodies may persist for 25 years or more. Further doses are not recommended. Serological testing to assess antibody levels after vaccination is not indicated. Given the long incubation period of hepatitis A (average 2–4 weeks), the vaccine can be administered up to the day of departure and still protect travellers. The use of immune globulin is now virtually obsolete for the purposes of travel prophylaxis.

A combination hepatitis A/typhoid (Vi CPS) vaccine, administered as a single dose, confers high levels of protection against both these waterborne diseases. A second dose of monovalent hepatitis A vaccine is needed 6–24 months later. (Boosters of typhoid vaccine should be given at 3-yearly intervals.)

A combination vaccine that provides protection against both hepatitis A and hepatitis B may be considered for travellers who may be exposed to both organisms. Primary immunization with the combined hepatitis A and B vaccine consist of three doses, given on a schedule of 0, 1 and 6 months. Alternatively, this combination vaccine may be administered on days 0, 7 and 21, with a booster dose at 12 months. Minor local and systemic reactions are fairly common. Minimum age is 1 year.

People born and raised in developing countries, and those born before 1945 in industrialized countries, have usually been HAV-infected in childhood and are likely to be immune. For such individuals, it may be cost-effective to test for antibodies to hepatitis A virus (anti-HAV) so that unnecessary vaccination can be avoided.

Type of vaccine:	Inactivated, given i.m.
Number of doses:	Two
Schedule:	Second dose 6–24 months after the first
Additional boosters:	May not be necessary
Contraindications:	Hypersensitivity to previous dose
Adverse reactions:	Mild local reaction of short duration, mild systemic reaction
Before departure:	Protection 2–4 weeks after first dose
Recommended for:	All non-immune travellers to countries or areas at risk
Special precautions:	None

HEPATITIS B

Cause	Hepatitis B virus (HBV), belonging to the Hepadnaviridae family.
Transmission	Infection is transmitted from person to person by contact with infected body fluids. Sexual contact is an important mode of transmission, but infection is also transmitted by transfusion of contaminated blood or blood products, or by use of contaminated needles or syringes for injections. There is also a potential risk of transmission through other skin-penetrating procedures, including acupuncture, piercing and tattooing. Perinatal transmission may occur from mother to baby. There is no insect vector or animal reservoir.
Nature of the disease	Most HBV infections are asymptomatic or cause mild symptoms, which are often unrecognized. Symptomatic disease occurs in about 1% of perinatally infected individuals, in 10% of children infected between 1 and 5 years of age, and in about 30% of individuals infected after the age of 5 years. Clinical hepatitis has a gradual onset, with anorexia, abdominal discomfort, nausea, vomiting, arthralgia and rash, followed by the development of jaundice in some cases. In adults, about 1% of cases are fatal. Chronic HBV infection develops in <5% of HBV-infected adults, but more often in young children and in the majority of those infected perinatally. In some cases of chronic HBV infection, cirrhosis and/or liver cancer develop later.
Disease burden	The endemicity of hepatitis B in a population is described by the prevalence of HBsAg, an HBV-specific component found in the blood (and other body fluids) in both acute and chronic stages of the infection. Hepatitis B is found worldwide, but with differing levels of risk. In certain areas of North America, northern and western Europe, the southern cone of South America, Australia and New Zealand, prevalence of chronic HBV infection is relatively low (less than 2% of the general population is HBsAg-positive) (Map).
Risk for travellers	The risk depends on (1) the prevalence of HBV infection in the country or area of destination, (2) the extent of direct contact with blood or body fluids or of sexual contact with potentially infected individuals, and (3) the duration

Hepatitis A, countries or areas at risk

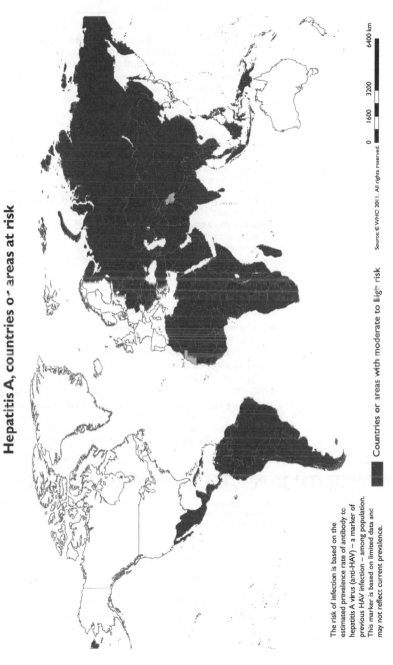

The risk of infection is based on the estimated prevalence rate of antibody to hepatitis A virus (anti-HAV) – a marker of previous HAV infection – among population. This marker is based on limited data and may not reflect current prevalence.

Countries or areas with moderate to high risk

0   1600   3200   6400 km

and type of travel. Principal risky activities include health care interventions (medical, dental, laboratory or other) that entail direct exposure to human blood or body fluids; receipt of a transfusion of blood that has not been tested for HBV; and exposure to needles (e.g. acupuncture, piercing, tattooing or injecting drug use) that have not been appropriately sterilized. In addition, transmission from HBV-positive to HBV-susceptible individuals may occur through direct contact between open skin lesions following a penetrating bite or scratch.

Precautions	The vaccine should be considered for all non-immune individuals travelling to countries or areas with moderate to high risk of infection. It can be administered to infants from birth. Also see Precautions under "HIV/AIDS and other sexually transmitted infections", Chapter 5.
Vaccine	Hepatitis B vaccine is produced by recombinant DNA technology, most commonly in yeast. The complete series consists of three doses of vaccine; the first two doses are usually given 1 month apart, with the third dose 1–12 months later. The WHO-recommended schedule for hepatitis B immunization of children consists of a dose within 24 h of birth followed by a second and third dose of hepatitis-B containing vaccines at intervals of at least 4 weeks.

A complete series of immunization provides protection for at least 15 years and, according to current scientific evidence, probably for life. Boosters are not recommended.

Because of the prolonged incubation period of hepatitis B, some protection will be afforded to most travellers following the second dose given before travel. However, the final dose should always be given.

A combination vaccine that provides protection against both hepatitis A and hepatitis B should be considered for travellers who may be exposed to both organisms. This inactivated vaccine is administered as follows: day 0; 1 month; 6 months. A rapid schedule of day 0, 1 month and 2 months with an additional dose at 12 months, and a very rapid schedule of day 0, day 7 and day 21 with a booster dose at 12 months, have been proposed by the vaccine manufacturer and approved by national regulatory authorities in some countries.

HUMAN PAPILLOMAVIRUS

Cause	Human papillomavirus (HPV), belonging to the Papillomaviridae family.
Transmission	Genital HPV infections are transmitted primarily by sexual contact, predominantly but not exclusively through penetrative intercourse. HPV is highly transmissible, and most sexually active men and women will acquire an HPV infection at some time in their lives.
Nature of the disease	Whereas most HPV infections are transient and benign, persistent genital infection with certain viral genotypes can lead to the development of anogenital precancers and cancers. Diseases caused by HPV include cancers of the cervix, vagina, vulva, penis and anus; a subset of head and neck cancers; anogenital warts; and recurrent respiratory papillomatosis.

Hepatitis B, countries or areas at risk

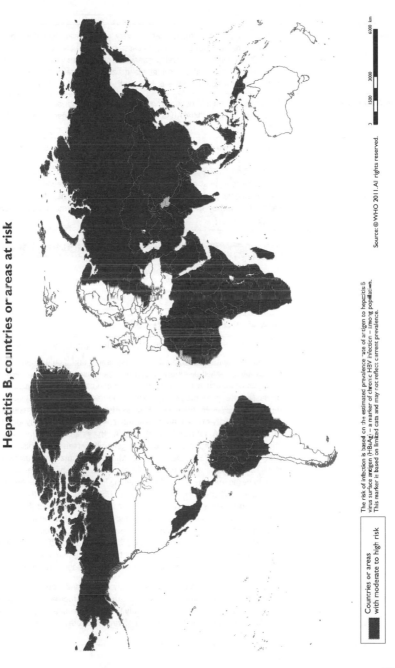

Countries or areas
with moderate to high risk

The risk of infection is based on the estimated prevalence rate of antigen to hepatitis B
virus surface antigen (HBsAg) – a marker of chronic HBV infection – among population.
This marker is based on limited data and may not reflect current prevalence.

0   1500   3000   6000 km

Disease burden	HPV is a family of viruses that are very common all over the world. In 2005, there were about 500 000 cases of cervical cancer worldwide and 260 000 related deaths. Cervical cancer incidence rates vary from 1 to 50 per 100 000 females; rates are highest in Latin America and the Caribbean, sub-Saharan Africa, Melanesia, and south-central and south-east Asia.
Risk for travellers	Transmission of HPV occurs most commonly through sexual activity; see precautions under "HIV/AIDS and other sexually transmitted infections" (Chapter 5).
Vaccines	Since 2006, two HPV vaccines have been licensed; one vaccine targets four and the other two HPV genotypes. Both vaccines are designed to protect against about 70% of cervical cancer cases worldwide (the 4-valent vaccine also protects against genital warts). The vaccines are intended for use primarily in adolescent girls aged 10–14 years. Over the next few years, HPV vaccination will be introduced into the immunization schedules of several countries.

INFLUENZA

AVIAN INFLUENZA

Chapter 5.

SEASONAL INFLUENZA AND INFLUENZA A (H1N1)

Cause	Influenza viruses belonging to the family Orthomyxoviridae.
	The influenza viruses are classified into types A, B and C on the basis of their core proteins. Only types A and B cause human disease of any concern. The subtypes of influenza A viruses are determined by envelope glycoproteins possessing either haemagglutinin (HA) or neuraminidase (NA) activity. High mutation rates and frequent genetic reassortments of these viruses contribute to great variability of the HA and NA antigens. All of the currently identified 16 HA and 9 NA subtypes of influenza A viruses are maintained in wild, aquatic bird populations. Humans are generally infected by viruses of the subtypes H1, H2 or H3, and N1 or N2. Minor point mutations causing small changes ("antigenic drift") occur relatively often. Antigenic drift enables the virus to evade immune recognition, resulting in repeated influenza outbreaks during interpandemic years. Major changes in the HA antigen ("antigenic shift") are caused by reassortment of genetic material from different A subtypes. Antigenic shifts resulting in new pandemic strains are rare events, occurring through reassortment between animal and human subtypes, for example in co-infected pigs. Influenza A (H1N1) virus emerged in 2009. It is a new reassortment that has never before circulated among humans. This virus is not closely related to previous or current human seasonal influenza viruses.
Transmission	Respiratory transmission occurs mainly by droplets disseminated by unprotected coughs and sneezes. Short-distance airborne transmission of influenza viruses may occur, particularly in crowded enclosed spaces. Hand contamination and direct inoculation of virus is another possible source of transmission.

Nature of the disease	An acute respiratory infection of varying severity, ranging from asymptomatic infection to fatal disease. Typical influenza symptoms include fever with abrupt onset, chills, sore throat, non-productive cough and, often accompanied by headache, coryza, myalgia and prostration. Complications of influenza viral infection include: primary influenza viral pneumonitis, bacterial pneumonia, otitis media and exacerbation of underlying chronic conditions. Illness tends to be most severe in the elderly, in infants and young children, and in immunocompromised hosts. Death resulting from seasonal influenza occurs mainly in the elderly and in individuals with pre-existing chronic diseases. Influenza A (H1N1) is similar to seasonal influenza but has been characterized by higher activity during the northern summer season, higher fatality rates among healthy young adults and higher incidence of viral pneumonia.
Disease burden	Influenza occurs all over the world, with an annual global attack rate estimated at 5–10% in adults and 20–30% in children. In temperate regions, influenza is a seasonal disease occurring typically in winter months: it affects the northern hemisphere from November to April and the southern hemisphere from April to September. In tropical areas there is no clear seasonal pattern, and influenza circulation is year-round, typically with several peaks during rainy seasons.
Risk for travellers	Travellers, like local residents, are at risk in any country during the influenza season. In addition, groups of travellers that include individuals from areas affected by seasonal influenza (e.g. cruise ships) may experience out-of-season outbreaks. Travellers visiting countries in the opposite hemisphere during the influenza season are at special risk, particular if they do not have some degree of immunity through recent infection or regular vaccination. The elderly, people with pre-existing chronic diseases and young children are most susceptible to complications.
Precautions	Whenever possible, avoid crowded enclosed spaces and close contact with people suffering from acute respiratory infections. Frequent hand-washing, especially after direct contact with ill persons or their environment, may reduce the risk of acquiring illness. Ill persons should be encouraged to practise cough etiquette (maintain distance, cover coughs and sneezes with disposable tissues or clothing, wash hands).
Vaccine	Influenza viruses constantly evolve, with rapid changes in their characteristics. To be effective, influenza vaccines need to stimulate immunity that protects against the principal strains of virus circulating at the time. Every year, the composition of influenza vaccines is modified separately for the northern and southern hemispheres. Since the antigenic changes in circulating influenza viruses can occur abruptly and at different times of the year, there may be significant differences between prevailing influenza strains in the northern and southern hemispheres. The internationally available vaccines contain three inactivated viral strains, the composition of which is modified every 6 months to ensure protection against the strains prevailing in each influenza season. The composition of vaccines is therefore adjusted for the hemisphere in which the vaccine will be used. Thus, a vaccine obtainable in one hemisphere may offer only partial protection against influenza infection in the other hemisphere, although in some years the viruses in the vaccine

may be antigenically identical. Available influenza vaccines do not protect against avian influenza.

Travellers with conditions that place them at high risk for complications of influenza should be vaccinated every year. In years in which the northern and southern hemisphere influenza vaccine strains differ, high-risk individuals travelling from one hemisphere to the other shortly before or during the other hemisphere's influenza season should obtain vaccination for the opposite hemisphere 2 weeks before travel. Where this is not possible, the traveller should arrange vaccination as soon as possible after arriving at the travel destination. During the 2010 season, a trivalent vaccine containing protection against influenza A (H1N1) was available in most countries.

Trivalent inactivated influenza vaccines are injected into the deltoid muscle (vaccinees aged >1 year) or the anterolateral aspect of the thigh (vaccinees aged 6–12 months). These vaccines should not be given to children under the age of 6 months; those aged 6–36 months should receive half the adult dose. Previously unvaccinated children aged less than 9 years should receive two injections, administered at least 1 month apart. A single dose of the vaccine is appropriate for schoolchildren aged 9 years and over and for healthy adults. Mild local reactions such as pain or swelling at the injection site are common; systemic reactions such as fever are less common. Vaccination is relatively contraindicated in case of egg allergy.

JAPANESE ENCEPHALITIS

Cause	Japanese encephalitis virus belongs to the mostly vector-borne Flaviviridae family.
Transmission	Pigs and various wild birds represent the natural reservoir of this virus, which is transmitted to new animal hosts and occasionally humans by mosquitoes of the genus *Culex*.
Nature of the disease	Most infections in humans are asymptomatic. In symptomatic cases, severity varies: mild infections are characterized by febrile headache or aseptic meningitis or encephalitis; severe cases have a rapid onset and progression with headache, high fever and meningeal signs. Permanent neurological sequelae are common among survivors. Approximately 25% of severe clinical cases have a fatal outcome.
Geographical distribution	Japanese encephalitis (JE) is the leading cause of viral encephalitis in Asia and occurs in almost all Asian countries (Map). Largely as a result of immunization, its incidence has been declining in Japan and the Republic of Korea and in some regions of China, but the disease is increasingly reported from Bangladesh, parts of India, Nepal, parts of Pakistan, northern Thailand and Viet Nam. Transmission occurs principally in rural agricultural locations where flooding irrigation is practised – some of which may be near or within urban centres. Transmission is mainly related to the rainy season in southeast Asia, but year-round transmission occurs, particularly in tropical climate zones. In the temperate regions of China, Japan, the Korean peninsula and eastern parts of the Russian Federation, transmission occurs mainly during the summer and autumn.

Risk for travellers	The risk for Japanese encephalitis is very low for most travellers to Asia, particularly for short-term visitors to urban areas, However, the risk varies according to season, destination, duration of travel and activities. Vaccination is recommended for travellers with extensive outdoor exposure (camping, hiking, working, etc.) during the transmission season in countries or areas at risk, particularly where flooding irrigation is practised. Whereas Japanese encephalitis in countries or areas at risk is primarily a disease of children, it can occur in travellers of any age. Prevention is by avoidance of mosquito bites (Chapter 3) and by vaccination.
Vaccine	The inactivated mouse-brain-derived (IMB) vaccine is now commonly replaced by cell-culture-based vaccines. The live attenuated SA 14-14-2 vaccine is widely used in China and in an increasing number of countries within the region. The product is not licensed or marketed outside the countries or areas at risk.

A new Vero cell-derived inactivated JE vaccine was approved in 2009 in North America, Australia and various European countries. The vaccine is inactivated, alum-adjuvanted, and based on the attenuated SA 14-14-2 JE viral strain. For the two-dose primary immunization, the manufacturer recommends intramuscular administration of the doses 4 weeks apart. The durability of protective immunity and the timing of a likely booster dose are still under investigation. This vaccine has been given concomitantly with hepatitis A vaccine without significant interference with safety and immunogenicity. Data on concomitant administration with other vaccines frequently used in travellers are currently unavailable. The vaccine is licensed for use in individuals 17 years of age and older in the United States, and 18 years and above in other countries. Post-marketing safety studies are under way.

The inactivated Vero cell JE vaccine (JE-VC) by BIKEN was licensed by the Japanese authorities in February 2009. JE-VC uses the same strain of JE virus (Beijing-1) as the mouse-brain-derived vaccine. Four clinical trials evaluating the safety and immunogenicity of JE-VC have been completed; seroconversion rates exceeded 95%. This vaccine is currently not available outside Japan.

Precautions and contraindications

A hypersensitivity reaction to a previous dose is a contraindication. The live attenuated vaccine should be avoided in pregnancy unless the likely risk favours its administration. Rare, but serious, neurological adverse events attributed to IMB vaccine have been reported from countries or areas at risk as well as from non-risk countries or areas. Allergic reactions to components of the vaccine occur occasionally. As such reactions may occur up to 2 weeks after administration, it is advisable to ensure that the complete course of vaccine is administered well in advance of departure.

Type of vaccine:	Inactivated mouse brain derived or live attenuated JE
Schedule:	For the inactivated vaccine: three doses at days 0, 7 and 28; or two doses given preferably 4 weeks apart (0.5 or 1.0 ml for adults, 0.25 or 0.5 ml for children, depending on the vaccines)

	For the live attenuated SA 14-14-2 vaccine equally good protection is achieved with a single dose
	Booster (IMB only): the duration of immunity after serial booster doses in adult travellers has not been well established for this vaccine. For children aged 1–3 years, the mouse-brain-derived vaccine provides adequate protection throughout childhood following two primary doses 4 weeks apart and boosters after 1 year and subsequently at 3-yearly intervals until the age of 10–15 years
Contraindications:	Hypersensitivity to a previous dose of vaccine, pregnancy and immunosuppression (live vaccine)
Adverse reactions:	Occasional mild local or systemic reaction; occasional severe reaction with generalized urticaria, hypotension and collapse
Before departure:	Inactivated vaccine, at least two doses before departure. Live attenuated vaccine, one dose is enough
Type of vaccine:	Inactivated, alum-adjuvanted, Vero cell-derived SA14-14-2 vaccine
Schedule:	2 intramuscular doses 4 weeks apart
Booster:	The timing of possible booster doses has not yet been established
Contraindications:	History of hypersensitivity to any component of the vaccine
Adverse reactions:	Occasional mild local or systemic reactions
Special precautions:	Safety and effectiveness have not been established in pregnant women, in nursing mothers, or in children and adolescents (younger than 17 years of age).
Before departure:	Immunization series should be completed at least 1 week before potential exposure to JEV.

Japanese encephalitis, countries or areas at risk, 2010

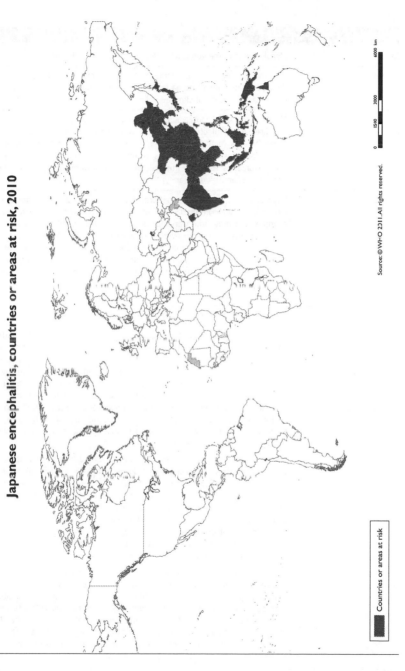

Countries or areas at risk

MEASLES

Cause	Measles virus of the genus *Morbillivirus* of the family Paramyxoviridae.
Transmission	Transmission, which is primarily by large respiratory droplets, increases during the late winter and early spring in temperate climates and after the rainy season in tropical climates.
Nature of the disease	Measles is a highly contagious infection; before vaccines became available, this disease had affected most people by the time of adolescence. Common complications include middle-ear infection and pneumonia. High-risk groups for measles complications include infants and individuals suffering from chronic diseases and impaired immunity, or from severe malnutrition (including vitamin A deficiency).
Disease burden	Measles occurs in a seasonal pattern. However, following the introduction of large-scale measles immunization, far fewer cases now occur in industrialized countries and indigenous transmission has virtually stopped in the Americas. Epidemics may still occur every 2 or 3 years in areas where there is low vaccine coverage. In countries where measles has been largely eliminated, cases imported from other countries remain an important continuing source of infection. In 2009, worldwide measles vaccination coverage had reached 82%, and between 2000 and 2008 the estimated annual number of deaths from measles dropped from 733 000 to 164 000.
Risk for travellers	Travellers who are not fully immunized against measles are at risk.
Vaccine	A number of live, attenuated measles vaccines are currently available, either as monovalent vaccine or as measles-containing vaccine combinations with one or more of rubella (R), mumps (M) and varicella vaccines. The measles/mumps/rubella (MMR) or measles/rubella (MR) vaccine is given in many countries instead of monovalent measles vaccine. The measles vaccines that are now internationally available are safe and effective and may be used interchangeably in immunization programmes. Every child should receive two doses of measles vaccine. The second dose may be given as early as 1 month following the first, depending on the local programmatic and epidemiological situation.
	Special attention must be paid to all children and adolescent/young adult travellers who have not received two doses of measles vaccine. Measles is still common in many countries and travel in densely populated areas may favour transmission. For infants travelling to countries experiencing extensive measles transmission, a dose of vaccine may be given as early as 6 months of age. However, children who receive the first dose between 6 and 8 months of age should subsequently receive the two doses according to the national schedule. Older children or adults who did not receive the two lifetime doses should consider measles vaccination before travel.
	Given the severe course of measles in patients with advanced HIV infection, measles vaccination should be routinely administered to potentially susceptible, asymptomatic HIV-positive children and adults. Measles vaccination may be considered even in individuals with symptomatic HIV infection, provided that they are not severely immunosuppressed. Where the risk of contracting measles infection is negligible, physicians who are able to monitor CD4 counts may prefer to delay the use of measles vaccine until

CD4 counts are above 200. Following measles vaccination no increased risk of serious adverse events has been demonstrated in HIV-positive compared with HIV-negative children, although lower antibody levels may be found in the former group.

MENINGOCOCCAL DISEASE

Cause	The bacterium *Neisseria meningitidis*. Most cases of meningococcal disease are caused by serogroups A, B and C; less commonly, infection is caused by serogroups Y (emerging in the United States) and W-135 (particularly in Saudi Arabia and west Africa) and rarely by serogroup X (Africa, Europe, United States).
Transmission	Transmission occurs by direct person-to-person contact and through respiratory droplets from the nose and pharynx of infected individuals, patients or asymptomatic carriers. Humans are the only reservoir.
Nature of the disease	Most infections do not cause clinical disease. Many infected people become asymptomatic carriers of the bacteria and serve as a reservoir and source of infection for others. In general, susceptibility to meningococcal disease decreases with age, although there is a small increase in risk in adolescents and young adults. Meningococcal meningitis has a sudden onset of intense headache, fever, nausea, vomiting, photophobia and stiff neck, plus various neurological signs. The disease is fatal in 5–10% of cases even with prompt antimicrobial treatment in good health care facilities, among individuals who survive, up to 20% have permanent neurological sequelae. Meningococcal septicaemia, in which there is rapid dissemination of bacteria in the bloodstream, is a less common form of meningococcal disease, characterized by circulatory collapse, haemorrhagic skin rash and high fatality rate.
Geographical distribution	Sporadic cases are found worldwide. In temperate zones, most cases occur in the winter months. Localized outbreaks occur in enclosed crowded spaces (e.g. dormitories, military barracks). In sub-Saharan Africa, in a zone stretching across the continent from Senegal to Ethiopia (the African "meningitis belt"), large outbreaks and epidemics take place during the dry season (November to June). Recent reports of group Y meningococcal disease in the United States, and outbreaks caused by serogroup W-135 strains in Saudi Arabia and sub-Saharan Africa, particularly Burkina Faso, suggest that these serogroups may be gaining in importance.
Risk for travellers	The risk of meningococcal disease in travellers is generally low. Those travelling to industrialized countries may be exposed to sporadic cases mostly of A, B or C. Outbreaks of meningococcal C disease occur in schools, colleges, military barracks and other places where large numbers of adolescents and young adults congregate.
	Travellers to the sub-Saharan meningitis belt may be exposed to outbreaks, most commonly of serogroup A and serogroup W135 disease, with comparatively very high incidence rates during the dry season (December to June). Long-term travellers living in close contact with the indigenous population may be at greater risk of infection.
	Pilgrims to Mecca are at particular risk. The tetravalent vaccine, (A, C, Y, W-135) is currently required by Saudi Arabia for pilgrims visiting Mecca for the Hajj (annual pilgrimage) or for the Umrah.

Precautions	Avoid overcrowding in confined spaces. Following close contact with an individual suffering from meningococcal disease, medical advice should be sought regarding possible chemoprophylaxis.
Vaccine	*Polysaccharide meningococcal vaccines*

Internationally marketed meningococcal polysaccharide vaccines are either bivalent (A and C) or tetravalent (A, C, Y and W-135).The vaccines are purified, heat-stable, lyophilized capsular polysaccharides from meningococci of the respective serogroups.

Both group A and group C vaccines have documented short-term efficacy levels of 85–100% in older children and adults. However, group C vaccines do not prevent disease in children under 2 years of age, and the efficacy of group A vaccine in children under 1 year of age is unclear. Group Y and W-135 polysaccharides have been shown to be immunogenic only in children over 2 years of age.

A protective antibody response occurs within 10 days of vaccination. In schoolchildren and adults, the bivalent and tetravalent polysaccharide vaccines appear to provide protection for at least 3 years, but in children under 4 years the levels of specific antibodies decline rapidly after 2–3 years.

The currently available bivalent and tetravalent meningococcal vaccines are recommended for immunization of specific risk groups as well as for large-scale immunization, as appropriate, for the control of meningococcal outbreaks caused by vaccine-preventable serogroups (A and C, or A, C, Y, W-135 respectively). Travellers who have access to the tetravalent polysaccharide vaccine (A, C, Y, W-135) should opt for this rather than the bivalent vaccine because of the additional protection against groups Y and W-135.

These vaccines do not provide any protection against group B meningococci, which are the leading cause of meningococcal disease in some countries.

Precautions and contraindications – polysaccharide vaccine

The internationally available polysaccharide vaccines are safe, and significant systemic reactions have been extremely rare. The most common adverse reactions are erythema and slight pain at the site of injection for 1–2 days. Fever exceeding 38.5 °C occurs in up to 2% of vaccinees. No significant change in safety or reactogenicity has been observed when the different group-specific polysaccharides are combined into bivalent or tetravalent meningococcal vaccines.

Type of vaccine:	Purified bacterial capsular polysaccharide meningococcal vaccine (bivalent or tetravalent)
Number of doses:	One
Duration of protection:	3–5 years
Contraindications:	Serious adverse reaction to previous dose
Adverse reactions:	Occasional mild local reactions; rarely, fever
Before departure:	2 weeks

Consider for:	All travellers to countries in the sub-Saharan meningitis belt and to areas with current epidemics; Hajj and Umrah pilgrims (required)
Special precautions:	Children under 2 years of age are not protected by the vaccine

Conjugate meningococcal vaccines

A T-cell-dependent immune response is achieved through conjugation of the polysaccharide to a protein carrier. Conjugate vaccines are therefore associated with an increased immunogenicity among infants and prolonged duration of protection.

Monovalent serogroup C conjugate vaccines were first licensed for use in 1999 and are now incorporated in national vaccination programmes in an increasing number of countries. In contrast to group C polysaccharide vaccines, the group C conjugate vaccine elicits adequate antibody responses and immunological memory even in infants who are vaccinated at 2, 3 and 4 months of age. Cross-protection does not occur and travellers already immunized with conjugate vaccine against serogroup C are not protected against other serogroups.

A tetravalent conjugate vaccine against serogroups A, C, Y, W-135 has been licensed in North America and some other countries. This vaccine is expected to induce protection of similar efficacy but longer duration compared to the polysaccharide tetravalent meningococcal vaccine

Precautions and contraindications – tetravalent conjugate meningococcal vaccine

Type of vaccine:	Conjugate vaccine against A, C, Y, and W135
Number of doses:	One
Duration of protection:	>3–5 years
Contraindications:	Serious adverse reaction to previous dose
Adverse reactions:	Occasional mild local reactions; rarely, fever
Before departure:	2 weeks
Consider for:	Travellers to countries in the sub-Saharan meningitis belt and to areas with current epidemics; Hajj and Umrah pilgrims
Special precautions:	Currently not licensed in the United States for children under age 2 and for individuals over 55 years of age

Meningococcal meningitis,* countries or areas at high risk, 2009

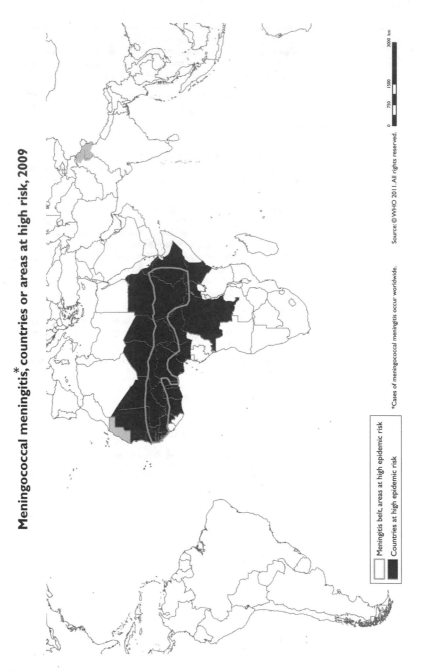

Meningitis belt, areas at high epidemic risk

Countries at high epidemic risk

*Cases of meningococcal meningitis occur worldwide.

0   750   1500   3000 km

MUMPS

Cause	Mumps virus of the genus *Rubulavirus* of the family Paramyxoviridae.
Transmission	Humans are the only known natural host for mumps virus, which is spread via direct contact or by airborne droplets from the upper respiratory tract of infected individuals.
Nature of the disease	Mumps (parotitis epidemica) is a viral infection of humans, primarily affecting the salivary glands. Although it is mostly a mild childhood disease, with peak incidence occurring among those aged 5–9 years, the mumps virus may also affect adults, among whom complications such as meningitis and orchitis are relatively more common. Encephalitis and permanent neurological sequelae are rare complications.
Disease burden	In most areas, annual mumps incidence is in the range of 100–1000 per 100 000 population, with epidemic peaks every 2–5 years. Natural infection with mumps virus is thought to confer lifelong protection.
Risk for travellers	Travellers who are not fully immunized against mumps are at risk.
Vaccine	The mumps vaccine is usually given in combination with measles and rubella vaccine (MMR). The attenuated strains of mumps virus that are currently used for the production of live mumps vaccines are all considered to be safe and efficacious. In order to avoid possible interference with persistent maternal antibodies, the first of the two recommended doses of the vaccine is usually given at 12–18 months of age. A single dose of mumps vaccine, either as single antigen or in combination, has a protective efficacy of 90–96%. The second dose provides protection to most individuals who did not respond to the first and should be given after a minimum interval of 1 month. In some countries the second dose is given at the age of 4–6 years.

PNEUMOCOCCAL DISEASE

Cause	The bacterium *Streptococcus pneumoniae*.
Transmission	Infection is acquired by direct person-to-person contact via respiratory droplets or oral contact. There are many healthy, asymptomatic carriers of the bacteria, but there is no animal reservoir or insect vector.
Nature of the disease	Pneumonia with empyema and/or bacteraemia, febrile bacteraemia and meningitis are the commonest manifestations of invasive pneumococcal infection. Pneumococci are a frequent cause of non-bacteraemic pneumonia. In developing countries, non-bacteraemic pneumonia causes the majority of pneumococcal deaths in children. Middle-ear infections, sinusitis and bronchitis are non-invasive and less severe manifestations of pneumococcal infection but are considerably more common. Several chronic conditions predispose to serious pneumococcal disease. Increasing pneumococcal resistance to antibiotics underlines the importance of vaccination.
Disease burden	Infection with pneumococcus is a major cause of morbidity and mortality worldwide. In 2005, WHO estimated that 1.6 million deaths were caused by this agent annually; this estimate included the deaths of 0.7–1 million children aged under 5 years. Most of these deaths occurred in poor coun-

tries and included a disproportionate number of children under the age of 2 years. In Europe and the USA, S. pneumoniae is the most common cause of community-acquired bacterial pneumonia in adults. In these regions, the annual incidence of invasive pneumococcal disease ranges from 10 to 100 cases per 100 000 population.

Risk for travellers

While travel itself does not normally increase the risk of acquiring pneumococcal disease, access to optimal health care may be limited during travel, increasing the risk of a poor outcome should disease occur. Certain conditions predispose to complications of pneumococcal infections, including sickle-cell disease, other haemoglobinopathies, chronic renal failure, chronic liver disease, immunosuppression after organ transplantation and other etiological factors, asplenia and dysfunctional spleen, leaks of cerebrospinal fluid, diabetes mellitus and HIV infection. Elderly individuals, especially those over 65 years of age, are also at increased risk for pneumococcal disease. Pneumococcal vaccine may be considered for travellers who belong to these high-risk groups.

Vaccine

A conjugate vaccine containing seven serotypes of the pneumococcus (PCV-7) is now available and is also safe and immunogenic in infants and children under 2 years of age. This vaccine is recommended by WHO as part of routine immunization in infants and has been introduced in some countries. It is advisable that children under 2 years of age (and high-risk children aged 2–5 years) are vaccinated against pneumococcal disease before undertaking travel. The primary series of PCV-7 consists of three intramuscular doses administered to infants at intervals of at least 4 weeks, starting at the age of 6 weeks or later. Some industrialized countries have adopted a schedule based on delivering two doses during infancy (for example, at 2 months and 4 months) and a third dose at 12–13 months. When the vaccine is initially introduced into childhood immunization programmes, a single catch-up dose of PCV-7 may be given to previously unvaccinated children aged 12–24 months and to children aged 2–5 years considered to be at high risk. This vaccine is licensed for children up to 5 years of age only.

In 2009, a 10-valent conjugated pneumococcal vaccine was licensed in Europe and is currently marketed in other parts of the world for use in children 6 weeks to 2 years of age. In addition to the pneumococcal components contained in the 7-valent vaccine, the 10-valent vaccine includes three components that ensure broader protection against the included invasive pneumococcal serotypes and also offer some protection against non-invasive infections, mainly otitis media (middle-ear infection).

In 2010, a 13-valent conjugated pneumococcal vaccine was licensed in the United States and is currently marketed internationally for immunization of children aged 6 weeks to 5 years for the prevention of invasive pneumococcal disease, as well as pneumonia and otitis media caused by these 13 pneumococcal serotypes.

The safety and reactogenicity profiles of the 10- and 13-valent vaccines are comparable to that of the 7-valent vaccine, and compatibility with major childhood vaccines has been demonstrated. The recommended primary vaccination schedule with both vaccines is three doses plus a booster.

The 23-valent polysaccharide vaccine (PPV23) represents pneumococcal serotypes that are responsible for 85–90% of invasive pneumococcal infections in the United States and some other industrialized countries. The vaccine is efficacious against invasive pneumococcal disease and pneumonia in otherwise healthy individuals, particularly young adults, but shows limited efficacy in this regard in other age groups, particularly young children; it is licensed only for individuals over 2 years of age. The 23-valent polysaccharide vaccine is commonly recommended for children and adults who have certain underlying medical conditions predisposing for pneumococcal infection, although its efficacy in several of these conditions is not well documented. In some countries, such as the United States, routine vaccination is recommended for everyone over 65 years of age. For primary immunization, PPV23 is administered as a single intramuscular dose (preferably in the deltoid muscle) or as a subcutaneous dose. The optimal timing, frequency and clinical effectiveness of additional doses of PPV23 are poorly defined, and national recommendations regarding revaccination vary. However, on the basis of the data on the duration of vaccine-induced protection, WHO suggests one single revaccination over 5 years of age after a first vaccination. Local adverse reactions may be more frequent in recipients of a second dose of PPV23 but are generally self-limiting and not severe.

POLIOMYELITIS (POLIO)

Cause	Poliovirus types 1, 2 and 3 (three closely related enteroviruses).
Transmission	In countries or areas reporting indigenous wild polio viruses the virus is spread predominantly by the faecal–oral route, although rare outbreaks caused by contaminated food or water have occurred. In settings with high standards of hygiene, the oral–oral route of transmission may also be common.
Nature of the disease	Poliomyelitis, also known as polio or infantile paralysis, is a disease of the central nervous system. After the virus enters the mouth, the primary site of infection is the intestine, although the virus can also be found in the pharynx. Fewer than 1% of those infected develop paralytic disease. In developing countries, 65–75% of cases currently occur in children under 3 years of age and 95% in children under 5 years of age. The resulting paralysis is permanent, although some recovery of function is possible. There is no cure.
Geographical distribution	Significant progress has been made towards global eradication of poliomyelitis. There are now (2010) only four countries where indigenous wild poliovirus (WPV) transmission has never been interrupted: Afghanistan, India, Nigeria and Pakistan (Map). Wild poliovirus importations from the four endemic countries into previously polio-free countries continue to occur, with some resulting in new outbreaks. As of late-2010, imported wild poliovirus was circulating in 14 previously polio-free countries: Angola, Chad, Democratic Republic of the Congo, Liberia, Mali, Mauritania, Nepal, Niger, Russian Federation, Senegal, Sierra Leone, Tajikistan, Turkmenistan and Uganda. Until wild poliovirus transmission has been stopped globally, all polio-free countries and areas remain at risk of importation and of renewed outbreaks.
Risk for travellers	The potential consequences of polio infection are crippling and sometimes life-threatening. Infection and paralysis may occur in non-immune individuals of any age. Infected travellers are potential vectors for transmission and possible reintroduction of the virus into polio-free zones. Until the disease has

been certified as eradicated globally, the risks of acquiring polio (for travellers to infected areas) and of reinfection of polio-free areas (by travellers from infected areas) remain. All travellers to and from countries or areas reporting wild polio virus should be adequately vaccinated. Updates on countries with ongoing transmission of indigenous and imported wild poliovirus and countries with recent transmission of imported wild poliovirus can be found at http://www.polioeradication.org/casecount.asp.

Vaccine

There are two types of vaccine: inactivated polio vaccine (IPV), which is given by injection, and oral polio vaccine (OPV), both based on polioviruses of serotypes 1, 2 and 3. IPV but not OPV is also marketed in combination with other vaccines.

OPV has been the vaccine of choice for controlling poliomyelitis in many countries because of its low cost, ease of administration and superiority in conferring intestinal immunity. On very rare occasions, however, OPV causes vaccine-associated paralytic poliomyelitis (VAPP). The risk of VAPP is higher with the first dose of OPV than with subsequent doses. VAPP is more common in individuals who are immunocompromised.

Most industrialized countries now use IPV, either as the sole vaccine against poliomyelitis or in schedules combined with OPV. Although IPV suppresses pharyngeal excretion of wild poliovirus, it has only limited effects in reducing intestinal excretion of poliovirus.

Following the first dose of polio vaccine, which is given at or shortly after birth (children at high risk of infection) or at 1–2 months of age (children at lower risk of infection), a second dose is administered 1–2 months later, with the third dose after 6–12 months. An additional dose is recommended after 4–6 years. For adults who have received a primary series of vaccination in childhood, a once-only additional dose is recommended in some countries. IPV is also the vaccine of choice to protect travellers to polio-infected areas who have no history of OPV use, as well as for immunocompromised individuals and their contacts and family members.

Travellers to countries or areas reporting indigenous wild polio viruses who have previously received three or more doses of OPV or IPV should be offered another dose of polio vaccine as a once-only dose before departure. Non-immunized individuals intending to travel to these countries or areas should complete a primary schedule of polio vaccination, using either IPV or OPV. For people who travel frequently to these countries or areas but stay for only brief periods, a once-only additional dose of a polio vaccine after the primary series should be sufficient to prevent disease.

Before travelling abroad, individuals living in countries or areas reporting indigenous wild polio viruses should have completed a full course of vaccination against polio, preferably with OPV, to boost mucosal immunity and reduce the risk of WPV shedding. Such travellers should receive an additional dose of OPV 1–12 months before each international journey.

In case of urgent travel, a minimum of one dose of OPV should be given, ideally 4 weeks before departure. Some polio-free countries (e.g. Saudi Arabia) may require travellers from countries or areas reporting wild polio viruses (see http://www.polioeradication.org/Dataandmonitoring/Poliothisweek.aspx) to be immunized against polio in order to obtain an entry visa, or they may require that travellers receive an additional dose on arrival, or both.

Polio affected countries for which WHO recommends polio immunization or boosting to travellers*

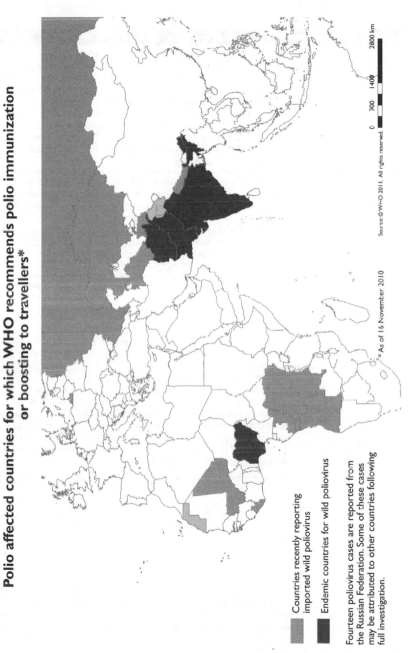

Countries recently reporting imported wild poliovirus

Endemic countries for wild poliovirus

Fourteen poliovirus cases are reported from the Russian Federation. Some of these cases may be attributed to other countries following full investigation.

* As of 16 November 2010

0   700   1400   2800 km

RABIES

Cause	The rabies virus, a lyssavirus of the family Rhabdoviridae.
Transmission	Rabies is a zoonotic disease affecting a wide range of domestic and wild mammals, including bats. Infection of humans usually occurs through the bite of an infected animal as the virus is present in the saliva. In developing countries, transmission is usually through dog bites. Transmission may occasionally also occur through other contact with a rabid animal, for example following a penetrating scratch with bleeding or licking of broken skin and mucosa. Person-to-person transmission other than via organ transplant has not been laboratory-confirmed.
Nature of the disease	An acute viral encephalomyelitis, which is almost invariably fatal. The initial signs include a sense of apprehension, headache, fever, malaise and sensory changes around the site of the animal bite. Excitability, hallucinations and abnormal fear of drafts of air (aerophobia) are common, followed in some cases by fear of water (hydrophobia) due to spasms of the swallowing muscles, progressing to delirium, convulsions and death a few days after onset. A less common form, paralytic rabies, is characterized by paralysis and loss of sensation, weakness and pain.
Disease burden	Rabies is present in mammals in many countries worldwide (Map). Most of the estimated 55 000 human rabies deaths per year occur in Africa and Asia. More information on rabies is available at http://www.who.int/rabies/rabnet/en.
Risk for travellers	The risk to travellers in areas countries and areas at risk for rabies (Map, or http://www.who.int/rabies/rabnet/en) is proportional to the probability of contact with potentially rabid mammals. In most developing countries, the estimated ratio of dogs, both owned and ownerless, to humans is 1:10 and an average 100 suspected rabid dog bites per 100 000 inhabitants are reported annually. According to a recent survey conducted in India, 1.6% of the total population received a dog bite during a 12-month period. As rabies is a lethal disease, medical advice should be sought immediately at a competent medical centre – ideally, the rabies treatment centre of a major city hospital. First-aid measures should also be started immediately (see "Post-exposure prophylaxis", below).
	Travellers should avoid contact with free-roaming animals, especially dogs and cats, and with wild, free-ranging and captive animals. For travellers who participate in caving or spelunking, casual exposure to cave air is not a concern, but cavers should be warned not to handle bats. In most countries of the world, suspect contact with bats should be followed by post-exposure prophylaxis.
	The map shows the WHO categories of risk, from no risk (rabies-free) countries or areas to countries or areas of low, medium and high risk (dog rabies). Categorization is based primarily on the animal host species in which the rabies virus is maintained in a country or area, e.g. bats and/or other wildlife and/or dogs and on the availability of reliable laboratory-based surveillance data in these reservoir species. Access to proper medical care and the availability of modern rabies vaccines have also been taken into consideration on a country basis. In countries or areas belonging to categories

2–4, pre-exposure immunization against rabies is recommended for travellers with certain characteristics:

Category 1: no risk.

Category 2: low risk. In these countries or areas travellers involved in activities that might bring them into direct contact with bats (for example, wildlife professionals, researchers, veterinarians and adventure travellers visiting areas where bats are commonly found) should receive pre-exposure prophylaxis.

Category 3: medium risk. In these countries or areas, travellers involved in any activities that might bring them into direct contact with bats and other wild animals, especially carnivores, (e.g., wildlife professionals, researchers, veterinarians and travellers visiting areas were bats and wildlife are commonly found) should receive pre-exposure prophylaxis.

Category 4: high risk. In these countries or areas, travellers spending a lot of time in rural areas involved in activities such as running, bicycling, camping or hiking should receive pre-exposure prophylaxis. Prophylaxis is also recommended for people with significant occupational risks, such as veterinarians, and expatriates living in areas with a significant risk of exposure to domestic animals, particularly dogs, and wild carnivores. Children should be immunized as they are at higher risk through playing with animals, particularly with dogs and cats; they may receive more severe bites and are less likely to report contact with suspect rabies animals.

Vaccine

Vaccination against rabies is used in two distinct situations:

- to protect those who are at risk of exposure to rabies, i.e. pre-exposure vaccination;

- to prevent the development of clinical rabies after exposure has occurred, usually following the bite of an animal suspected of having rabies, i.e. post-exposure prophylaxis.

The vaccines used for pre-exposure and post-exposure vaccination are the same, but the immunization schedule differs. Rabies immunoglobulin is used only for post-exposure prophylaxis. Modern vaccines of cell-culture or embryonated-egg origin are safer and more effective than the older vaccines, which were produced in brain tissue. These modern rabies vaccines are now available in major urban centres of most countries of the developing world. Rabies immunoglobulin, on the other hand, is in short supply worldwide and may not be available, even in major urban centres, in many dog rabies-infected countries.

Pre-exposure vaccination

Pre-exposure vaccination should be offered to people at high risk of exposure to rabies, such as laboratory staff working with rabies virus, veterinarians, animal handlers and wildlife officers, and other individuals living in or travelling to countries or areas at risk. Travellers with extensive outdoor exposure in rural areas – such as might occur while running, bicycling, hiking, camping, backpacking, etc. – may be at risk, even if the duration of travel is short. Pre-exposure vaccination is advisable for children living in or visiting countries or areas at risk, where they provide an easy target for rabid animals. Pre-exposure vaccination is also recommended for individuals travelling to isolated areas or to areas where immediate access to appropriate medical care is limited or to countries or areas where modern rabies vaccines are in short supply and locally available rabies vaccines might be unsafe and/or ineffective.

Pre-exposure rabies vaccination consists of three full intramuscular doses of cell-culture- or embryonated-egg-based vaccine given on days 0, 7 and 21 or 28 (a few days' variation in the timing is not important). For adults, the vaccine should always be administered in the deltoid area of the arm; for young children (under 1 years of age), the anterolateral area of the thigh is recommended. Rabies vaccine should never be administered in the gluteal area: administration in this manner will result in lower neutralizing antibody titres.

To reduce the cost of cell-derived vaccines for pre-exposure rabies vaccination, intradermal vaccination in 0.1-ml volumes on days 0, 7 and either 21 or 28 may be considered. This method of administration is an acceptable alternative to the standard intramuscular administration, but it is technically more demanding and requires appropriate staff training and qualified medical supervision. As an open vial should not be kept for more than 6 h, wastage can be avoided by vaccinating several people during that period. Concurrent use of chloroquine can reduce the antibody response to intradermal application of cell-culture rabies vaccines. People who are currently receiving malaria prophylaxis or who are unable to complete the entire three-dose pre-exposure series before starting malarial prophylaxis should therefore receive pre-exposure vaccination by the intramuscular route.

Rabies vaccines will induce long-lasting memory cells, giving rise to an accelerated immune response when a booster dose of vaccine is administered. Periodic booster injections are therefore not recommended for general travellers. However, *in the event of exposure through the bite or scratch of an animal known or suspected to be rabid, individuals who have previously received a complete series of pre- or post-exposure rabies vaccine (with cell-culture or embryonated-egg vaccine) should receive two booster doses of vaccine. Ideally, the first dose should be administered on the day of exposure and the second 3 days later.* This should be combined with thorough wound treatment (see "Post-exposure prophylaxis", below). Rabies immunoglobulin is not required for previously vaccinated patients. Periodic booster injections are recommended only for people whose occupations put them at continuous or frequent risk of rabies exposure, e.g. rabies researchers or staff in diagnostic laboratories where rabies virus is present. For more information on continuous or frequent risk, see WHO Expert Consultation on Rabies. For individuals at continuous or frequent risk of rabies exposure who have previously received pre-exposure rabies vaccination, a booster vaccination is administered if the serological titre falls below 0.5 IU/ml, the antibody level considered to be protective.

Precautions and contraindications

Modern rabies vaccines are well tolerated. The frequency of minor adverse reactions (local pain, erythema, swelling and pruritus) varies widely from one report to another. Occasional systemic reactions (malaise, generalized aches and headaches) have been noted after both intramuscular and intradermal injections.

Type of vaccine:	Modern cell-culture or embryonated-egg vaccine
Number of doses:	Three, one on each of days 0, 7 and 21 or 28, given i.m. (1 or 0.5 ml/dose depending on the vaccine) or i.d. (0.1 ml/ inoculation site)[a]
Booster:	Not routinely needed for general travellers[b]
Adverse reactions:	Minor local or systemic reactions
Before departure:	Pre-exposure prophylaxis for those planning a visit to a country or area at risk, especially if the area to be visited is far from major urban centres and appropriate care, including the availability of post-exposure rabies prophylaxis, cannot be assured.

[a] For information on which vaccines are recommended for intradermal use, see: http://www.who.int/rabies/human/postexp/en/index.html.

[b] In the event of exposure through the bite or scratch of an animal known or suspected to be rabid, individuals who have previously received a complete series of pre-exposure or post-exposure cell-culture or embryonated-egg rabies vaccine should receive two booster doses of vaccine, the first dose ideally on the day of exposure and the second 3 days later. Rabies immunoglobulin should not be administered.

Post-exposure prophylaxis

In countries or areas at risk of rabies, the circumstances of an animal bite or other contact with an animal suspected to be rabid may require post-exposure prophylaxis. In such situations, medical advice should be obtained immediately.

Strict adherence to the WHO-recommended guidelines for optimal post-exposure rabies prophylaxis virtually guarantees protection from the disease. The administration of vaccine, and immunoglobulin if required, must be conducted by, or under the direct supervision of, a physician. Post-exposure prophylaxis depends on the type of contact with the confirmed or suspect rabid animal, as follows:

Type of contact, exposure and recommended post-exposure prophylaxis

Category	Type of contact with a suspected or confirmed rabid domestic or wild[a] animal or animal unavailable for testing	Type of exposure	Recommended post-exposure prophylaxis
I	Touching or feeding of animals	None	None, if reliable case history is available
	Licks on intact skin		

[a] Exposure to rodents, rabbits and hares seldom, if ever, requires specific anti-rabies post-exposure prophylaxis.

II	Nibbling of uncovered skin Minor scratches or abrasions without bleeding	Minor	Administer vaccine immediately.[b] Stop treatment if animal remains healthy throughout an observation period of 10 days[c] or is proved to be negative for rabies by a reliable laboratory using appropriate diagnostic techniques
III	Single or multiple transdermal bites or scratches, licks on broken skin Contamination of mucous membrane with saliva (i.e. licks) Exposures to bats[d]	Severe	Administer rabies immunoglobulin and vaccine immediately. Stop treatment if animal remains healthy throughout an observation period of 10 days[c] or is proved to be negative for rabies by a reliable laboratory using appropriate diagnostic techniques

[b] If an apparently healthy dog or cat in or from a low-risk country or area is placed under observation, the situation may warrant delaying initiation of treatment.

[c] This observation period applies only to dogs and cats. Except in the case of threatened or endangered species, other domestic and wild animals suspected to be rabid should be humanely killed and their tissues examined for the presence of rabies antigen using appropriate laboratory techniques.

[d] Post-exposure prophylaxis should be considered for individuals who have been in close contact with bats, particularly following bites or scratches or exposure to mucous membranes.

1. Wound treatment

Thorough washing of the wound with soap/detergent and water, followed by the application of ethanol or an aqueous solution of iodine or povidone.

2. Passive immunization

Human rabies immunoglobulin (HRIG) or equine rabies immunoglobulin (ERIG) or F(ab')2 products for category III exposures as well as some category II exposures (see table, above). Passive immunization should be administered just before or shortly after administration of the first dose of vaccine given in the post-exposure prophylaxis regimen. If it is not immediately available, passive immunization can be administered up until the seventh day after initiation of the primary series of post-exposure prophylaxis (with cell-culture or embryonated-egg rabies vaccine).

Dosage and administration: The dose for HRIG is 20 IU/kg body weight and for ERIG and F(ab')2 products 40 IU/kg body weight. The full dose of rabies immunoglobulin, or as much as is anatomically feasible, should be administered into and around the wound site. Any remainder should be injected i.m. at a site distant from the site of active vaccine administration. Multiple needle injections into the wound should be avoided. If the correct dose of rabies immunoglobulin is too small to infiltrate all wounds, as might be true of a severely bitten individual, it can be diluted in physiological buffered saline to ensure greater wound coverage.

3. Active immunization

Cell-culture- or embryonated-egg-based rabies vaccines should always be used for post-exposure prophylaxis. They can be administered either i.m. or i.d.

Intramuscular regimens: Both a five-dose and a four-dose i.m. regimen are recommended for post-exposure vaccination; the five-dose ("Essen") regimen is the more commonly used:

- The five-dose ("Essen") regimen is administered on days 0, 3, 7, 14 and 28 into the deltoid muscle.

- The four-dose ("Zagreb") regimen is administered as two doses on day 0 (one dose in the right and one in the left deltoid), and then one dose on each of days 7 and 21 into the deltoid muscle.

An alternative post-exposure regimen for healthy, fully immunocompetent exposed people who receive wound care plus high quality rabies immu noglobulin plus WHO-prequalified rabies vaccines consists of four doses administered i.m. on days 0, 3, 7 and 14.

Intradermal regimens: Intradermal administration of cell-culture- and em-bryonated-egg-based rabies vaccines has been successfully used in many developing countries that cannot afford the five- or four-dose i.m. schedu-les.

- The two-site i.d. method: one i.d. injection at two sites on days 0, 3, 7 and 28.

For use with: 0.1 ml for purified Vero cell rabies vaccine (PVRV) (VerorabTM); 0.1 ml for purified chick embryo rabies vaccine (RabipurTM).

ROTAVIRUS

Cause	Rotaviruses, which belong to the family Reoviridae.
Transmission	Transmission is primarily by the faecal–oral route, directly from person to person or indirectly via contaminated fomites. A respiratory mode of trans-mission has also been proposed.
Nature of the disease	Rotavirus causes an acute gastroenteritis in infants and young children and is associated with profuse watery diarrhoea, projectile vomiting and fever. Rapid dehydration can occur, especially in very young infants, requiring rehydration therapy. The virus replicates in the enterocytes of the small intestine, causing extensive damage to the microvilli that results in malabsorption and loss of fluids and electrolytes.
Disease burden	Rotaviruses are found worldwide. They are the leading cause of severe, dehydrating diarrhoea in children under 5 years globally: outpatient visits are estimated at more than 25 million and hospitalizations attributable

Rabies, countries or areas at risk

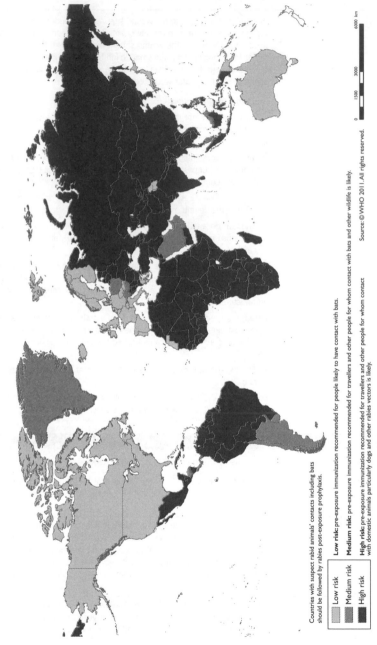

Countries with suspect rabid animals' contacts including bats should be followed by rabies post-exposure prophylaxis.

Low risk: pre-exposure immunization recommended for people likely to have contact with bats.

Medium risk: pre-exposure immunization recommended for travellers and other people for whom contact with bats and other wildlife is likely.

High risk: pre-exposure immunization recommended for travellers and other people for whom contact with domestic animals particularly dogs and other rabies vectors is likely.

Low risk
Medium risk
High risk

	to rotavirus infections at more than 2 million each year. Fatal outcomes, estimated in 2004 to be 527 000 (475 000–580 000) annually, occur predominantly in low-income countries. In temperate climates, the incidence of rotavirus gastroenteritis typically peaks during the winter season, whereas in tropical settings rotavirus occurs year round. Reinfection of older children and adults is common, although the infection is usually sub-clinical.
Risk for travellers	The potential risk for adult travellers is extremely limited since most individuals will have good immunity through repeated exposures early in life. Children under the age of 5 years are at risk.
Vaccine	Two live, attenuated, oral rotavirus vaccines are internationally licensed and routine childhood vaccination has been initiated in a number of countries. The clinical efficacy of the rotavirus vaccines has been demonstrated in most parts of the world. WHO recommends the inclusion of rotavirus vaccination in all national immunization programmes, particularly in countries or areas at risk. The first dose of either RotaTeq™ or Rotarix™ should be administered at 6–15 weeks of age, with an interval between doses of at least 4 weeks. The Rotarix™ vaccine is administered orally in a two-dose schedule while RotaTeq™ is administered orally in a three-dose schedule. With both vaccines, all doses should be administered before the age of 32 weeks. Vaccination is not currently recommended for travellers or older children outside the routine childhood immunization schedule.

RUBELLA

Cause	The rubella virus, a togavirus of the genus *Rubivirus*.
Transmission	Rubella virus is transmitted by the respiratory route and the virus replicates in the nasopharyngeal mucosa and local lymph nodes. Humans are the only known host.
Nature of the disease	Acquired rubella is characterized by a transient, erythematous rash, conjunctivitis, coryza, postauricular and suboccipital lymphadenopathy, low fever and nausea. Arthralgia and arthritis rarely occur in children, but may affect up to 70% of adults, particularly women. Haemorrhagic manifestations, Guillain–Barré syndrome and encephalitis are rarely reported. Serological studies have shown that 20–50% of all rubella infections are subclinical. Congenital rubella infection and congenital rubella syndrome (CRS) are caused by infection in early pregnancy. From just before conception and during the first 8–10 weeks of gestation, rubella infection may result in multiple fetal defects in up to 90% of cases and often causes miscarriage or stillbirth. Although the worldwide burden of CRS is not well characterized, it is estimated that more than 100 000 cases occur each year in developing countries alone.
Geographical distribution	Worldwide.
Risk for travellers	Travellers who are not immunized against rubella may be at risk when visiting countries where the vaccine coverage is suboptimal. Particular attention should be paid to ensuring protection of women who may become pregnant during the period of travel.

Vaccine	The internationally licensed rubella vaccines, based on live attenuated RA 27/3 strain of the rubella virus and propagated in human diploid cells, have proved safe and efficacious, achieving 95–100% protection, possibly lifelong, after just one dose. Following well-designed and well-implemented programmes using such vaccines, rubella and CRS have almost disappeared from many countries. Other attenuated vaccine strains are available in China and Japan.
	Rubella vaccine is commercially available in a monovalent form, in a bivalent combination with either measles or mumps vaccine, and in the trivalent measles/mumps/rubella (MMR) vaccine and other combinations. Rubella-containing vaccines are usually administrated at 12–15 months of age but may be offered to children as young as 9 months.
	Rubella vaccination of pregnant women should be avoided, and pregnancy should be avoided within 1 month of receiving the vaccine due to the theo-retical, but never demonstrated, risk of vaccine-induced CRS.

TICK-BORNE ENCEPHALITIS

Cause	The tick-borne encephalitis (TBE) virus of the family Flaviviridae. Three subtypes of the causative agent are known: the European, the Far Eastern (spring-summer encephalitis) and the Siberian. Other closely related viruses cause similar diseases.
Transmission	Infection is transmitted by the bite of infected ticks or occasionally by inges-tion of unpasteurized milk. There is no direct person-to-person transmission. Some related viruses, also tick-borne, infect animals such as birds, deer (louping-ill), rodents and sheep.
Nature of the disease	Infection may induce an influenza-like illness, with a second phase of fever occurring in 10% of cases. Encephalitis develops during the second phase and may result in paralysis, permanent sequelae or death. Severity of illness increases with age of the patient. The far-eastern subtype is believed to cause more severe symptoms and sequelae than the European subtype.
Geographical distribution	The European subtype is present in large parts of central and eastern Eu-rope, particularly Austria, southern Germany and northern Switzerland, the Baltic states (Estonia, Latvia, Lithuania), the Czech Republic, Hungary and Poland; the far-eastern subtype is found from north-eastern Europe to China and Japan, and the Siberian subtype from northern Europe to Siberia. The disease is seasonal; most cases occur during April to November. The risk is highest in forested areas up to an altitude of about 1400 m.
Risk for travellers	Travellers during the summer months in countries or areas at risk, are par-ticularly at risk when hiking or camping in rural or forested areas.
Precautions	Avoid bites by ticks by wearing long trousers and closed footwear when hiking or camping in countries or areas at risk. If a bite occurs, the tick should be removed as soon as possible.
Vaccine	The vaccine should be offered only to at-risk travellers. Two vaccines are available in Western Europe, in adult and paediatric formulations, based on the European subtype. These are inactivated vaccines containing a sus-

pension of purified TBE virus grown on chick embryo cells and inactivated with formaldehyde. Both provide safe and reliable protection. Immunity is induced against all subtypes of the TBE virus. Two doses of 0.5 ml should be given i.m. 4–12 weeks apart. A third dose is given 9–12 months after the second and confers immunity for at least 3 years. Booster doses are required to maintain immunity and should be given every 3–5 years if the risk continues. Outside countries or areas at risk, the vaccines may not be licensed and will have to be obtained by special request. In the Russian Federation, two locally produced inactivated vaccines are available that are based on the Far Eastern subtype.

Precautions and contraindications

Occasional local reactions may occur, such as reddening and swelling around the injection site, swelling of the regional lymph nodes or general reactions (e.g. fatigue, pain in the limb, nausea and headache). Rarely, there may be fever above 38 °C for a short time, vomiting or transient rash. In very rare cases, neuritis of varying severity may be seen, although the etiological relationship to vaccination is uncertain.

Type of vaccine:	Killed
Number of doses:	Two, given i.m. 4–12 weeks apart
Booster:	9–12 months after second dose and then every 3 years if risk of exposure persists
	Accelerated schedules for travellers: Depending on choice of TBE vaccine, the manufacturer recommends either a rapid schedule based on immunization on day 0, day 14 and month 5–7, or an accelerated schedule based on immunization on day 0, day 7 and day 21
Contraindications:	Hypersensitivity to the vaccine preservative thiomersal; adverse reaction to previous dose
Adverse reactions:	Local reactions occasionally; rarely fever
Before departure:	Second dose 2 weeks before departure
Recommended for:	High-risk individuals only
Special precautions:	Avoid ticks; remove ticks immediately if bitten

TUBERCULOSIS (TB)

Cause	*Mycobacterium tuberculosis*, the tubercle bacillus.
Transmission	Infection is usually by direct airborne transmission from person to person.
Nature of the disease	Exposure to *M. tuberculosis* may lead to infection, but most infections do not lead to disease. The risk of developing disease following infection is generally 5–10% during the lifetime but may be increased by various factors, notably immunosuppression (e.g. advanced HIV infection).

	Multidrug resistance refers to strains of *M. tuberculosis* that are resistant to at least isoniazid and rifampicin (MDR-TB). The resistant strains do not differ from other strains in infectiousness, likelihood of causing disease, or general clinical effects; if they do cause disease, however, treatment is more difficult and the risk of death will be higher. Extensively drug-resistant TB (XDR-TB) is TB that is resistant to at least isoniazid and rifampin, to any fluoroquinolone and to at least one of the injectable second-line anti-TB drugs capreomycin, kanamycin and amikacin.
Geographical distribution	Worldwide. The risk of infection differs between countries, as shown on the map of estimated tuberculosis incidence.
Risk for travellers	Most travellers are at low risk for TB. The risk for long-term (over 3 months) travellers in a country with a higher incidence of TB than their own may be comparable to the risk for local residents. Living conditions, as well as duration of travel and purpose of travel, e.g. emergency relief, are important in determining the risk of infection: high-risk settings include impoverished communities, areas experiencing civil unrest or war, refugee areas, health facilities, prisons and shelters for the homeless. Individuals with HIV infection are at higher risk of TB.
Precautions	Travellers should avoid close contact with known TB patients. For travellers from low-incidence countries who may be exposed to infection in relatively high-incidence countries (e.g. health professionals, humanitarian relief workers, missionaries), a baseline tuberculin skin test is advisable for comparison with retesting after return. If the skin reaction to tuberculin suggests recent infection, the traveller should receive, or be referred for, treatment for latent infection. Patients under treatment for TB should not travel until the treating physician has documented, by laboratory examination of sputum, that they are not infectious and are therefore of no risk to others. The importance of completing the prescribed course of treatment should be stressed.
Vaccine	All versions of the BCG vaccine are based on live, attenuated mycobacterial strains descended from the original, attenuated bacillus Calmette–Guérin. The vaccine is administered intradermally and can be given simultaneously with other childhood vaccines. BCG vaccine is contraindicated for individuals with severely impaired immunity and individuals with HIV infection.

BCG vaccine is of very limited use for travellers. In the first year of life it provides good protection against severe forms of TB (miliary TB and meningitis). In countries with high TB prevalence, infants are generally immunized with a single dose of BCG as soon after birth as possible. Children who are known to be HIV-infected, even if asymptomatic, should not be immunized with BCG vaccine. Other protective benefits of the vaccine are uncertain. One dose of BCG should be considered for unvaccinated infants travelling from an area of low incidence to one of high incidence.

Many industrialized countries with a low incidence of TB have ceased giving BCG routinely to neonates.

Booster doses of BCG are not recommended by WHO. |

Tuberculosis, estimated new cases, 2009

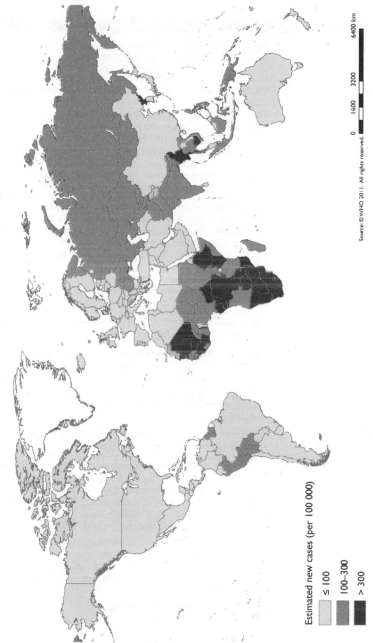

Estimated new cases (per 100 000)

≤ 100

100–300

> 300

0   1600   3200   6400 km

TYPHOID FEVER

Cause	*Salmonella typhi*, the typhoid bacillus, which infects only humans. Paratyphoid and enteric fevers are caused by other species of *Salmonella*, which infect domestic animals as well as humans.
Transmission	Infection is transmitted by consumption of contaminated food or water. Occasionally direct faecal–oral transmission may occur. Shellfish taken from sewage-polluted areas are an important source of infection. Infection occurs also through eating raw fruit and vegetables fertilized by night soil, and through ingestion of contaminated milk and milk products. Flies may cause human infection through transfer of the infectious agents to foods. Pollution of water sources may produce epidemics of typhoid fever, when large numbers of people use the same source of drinking-water.
Nature of the disease	A systemic disease of varying severity. Severe cases are characterized by gradual onset of fever, headache, malaise, anorexia and insomnia. Constipation is more common than diarrhoea in adults and older children. Without treatment, the disease progresses with sustained fever, bradycardia, hepatosplenomegaly, abdominal symptoms and, in some cases, pneumonia. In white-skinned patients, pink spots, which fade on pressure, appear on the skin of the trunk in up to 20% of cases. In the third week, untreated cases may develop gastrointestinal and other complications, which may prove fatal. Around 2–5% of those who contract typhoid fever become chronic carriers, as bacteria persist in the biliary tract after symptoms have resolved.
Geographical distribution	There is a higher risk of typhoid fever in countries or areas with low standards of hygiene and water supply facilities.
Risk for travellers	The risk for travellers is generally low, except in parts of northern and western Africa, in southern Asia, in parts of Indonesia and in Peru. Elsewhere, travellers are usually at risk only when exposed to low standards of hygiene. Even vaccinated travellers should take care to avoid consumption of potentially contaminated food and water as the vaccine does not confer 100% protection.
Precautions	Observe all precautions against exposure to foodborne and waterborne infections (Chapter 3).
Vaccine	• Oral Ty21a. The live, attenuated mutant strain of *Salmonella typhi* Ty21a, supplied in enteric coated capsules, is given in three doses (four in North America) 2 days apart. Protection is induced 7 days after the final dose. Seven years after the final dose the average protective efficacy was shown to be 67% in residents of countries or areas at risk but may be less effective in travellers. A liquid formulation is no longer available. • Injectable Vi CPS. The Vi polysaccharide vaccine (Vi CPS) contains 25 µg of polysaccharide per dose, and is given i.m. in a single dose. Protection is induced about 7 days after the injection. In countries or areas at risk, the protective efficacy after vaccination is about 72% after 1.5 years and 50% after 3 years. Both typhoid vaccines are safe and effective. A combined typhoid/hepatitis A vaccine is also available in some countries.

Precautions and contraindications

Proguanil, mefloquine and antibiotics should be stopped from 3 days before until 3 days after Ty21a is given.

No serious adverse effects have been reported following administration of Ty21a or Vi CPS.

These vaccines are not recommended for use in infant immunization programmes due to insufficient information on their efficacy in children under 2 years of age.

Type of vaccine:	Oral Ty21a and injectable Vi CPS
Number of doses:	Three or four doses of live Ty21a, given orally at 2-day intervals as enteric coated capsule. One dose of Vi CPS, given i.m.
Booster:	Every 2–3 years for Vi CPS; for Ty21a, see package insert.[a]
Contraindications:	There are no contraindications to the use of these vaccines other than previous severe hypersensitivity reaction to vaccine components.
Adverse reactions:	None significant
Before departure:	1 week
Recommended for:	Travellers to high-risk countries or areas and travellers staying longer than 1 month or likely to consume food or beverages away from the usual tourist routes in developing countries. Vaccination is particularly appropriate in countries or areas at risk where antibiotic-resistant strains of S. typhi are prevalent.
Special precautions:	Vi CPS – not under 2 years of age; avoid proguanil, mefloquine and antibiotics with Ty21a

[a] The duration of protection following Ty21a immunization is not well defined and may vary with vaccine dose and possibly with subsequent exposures to Salmonella typhi (natural booster). In Australia and Europe, 3 tablets are given on days 1, 3, and 5; this series is repeated every year for individuals travelling from non-endemic to endemic countries, and every 3 years for individuals living in countries or areas at risk. In North America, 4 tablets are given on days 1, 3, 5, and 7 and revaccination is recommended only after 7 years (Canada) or 5 years (USA) for all, regardless of typhoid fever risk in the country or area of residence.

VARICELLA

Cause	Varicella zoster virus (VZV), a herpesvirus belonging to the sub-family of Alphaherpesviridae.
Transmission	Transmission is via droplets, aerosol or direct contact, and patients are usually contagious from a few days before onset of the rash until the rash has crusted over.

Nature of the disease	Varicella (chickenpox) is an acute, highly contagious disease. In temperate climates most cases occur before the age of 10 years. The epidemiology is less well understood in tropical areas, where a relatively large proportion of adults in some countries are seronegative. While mostly a mild disorder in childhood, varicella tends to be more severe in adults. It is characterized by an itchy, vesicular rash, usually starting on the scalp and face, initially accompanied by fever and malaise. As the rash gradually spreads to the trunk and extremities, the first vesicles dry out. It normally takes about 7–10 days for all crusts to disappear. The disease may be fatal, especially in neonates and immunocompromised individuals. Complications include VZV-induced pneumonitis or encephalitis and invasive group A streptococcal infections. Following infection, the virus remains latent in neural ganglia; upon subsequent reactivation, VZV may cause zoster (shingles), a disease affecting mainly immunocompromised individuals and the elderly.
Geographical distribution	Worldwide.
Risk for travellers	In several industrialized countries, varicella vaccines have been introduced into the childhood immunization programmes. Most adult travellers from temperate climates are immune (as a result of either natural disease or immunization). Adult travellers without a history of varicella who travel from tropical countries to temperate climates may be at increased risk and should consider vaccination.
Vaccine	Various formulations of the live attenuated vaccine, based on the so-called Oka strain of VZV, are in use. Some formulations are approved for use in about 95% of healthy children. From both a logistic and an epidemiological point of view, the optimal age for varicella vaccination is 12–24 months. In some countries, one dose of the vaccine is considered sufficient, regardless of age. In the United States, two doses, 4–8 weeks apart, are recommended for adolescents and adults. In a few cases (<5%), vaccinees experience a mild varicella-like disease with rash within 4 weeks. Contraindications to varicella vaccine are pregnancy (because of a theoretical risk to the fetus; pregnancy should be avoided for 4 weeks following vaccination), ongoing severe illness, a history of anaphylactic reactions to any component of the vaccine, and immunosuppression.

YELLOW FEVER

Cause	The yellow fever virus, an arbovirus of the *Flavivirus* genus.
Transmission	Yellow fever occurs in urban and rural areas of Africa and central South America. In jungle and forest areas, monkeys are the main reservoir of infection, which is spread by mosquitoes from monkey-to-monkey and, occasionally, to humans. These mosquitoes bite during daylight hours. In urban settings mosquitoes transmit the virus from human-to-human and introduction of infection into densely populated urban areas can lead to large epidemics of yellow fever. In Africa, an intermediate pattern of transmission is common in humid savannah regions where mosquitoes infect both monkeys and humans, causing localized outbreaks.
Nature of the disease	Although most infections are asymptomatic, some lead to an acute illness characterized by two phases. Initially, there is fever, muscular pain, headache,

chills, anorexia, nausea and/or vomiting, often with bradycardia. About 15% of patients progress to a second phase after a few days, with resurgence of fever, development of jaundice, abdominal pain, vomiting and haemorrhagic manifestations; up to half of these patients die 10–14 days after the onset of illness.

Geographical distribution	Tropical areas of Africa and South America (Map). Transmission can occur at altitudes up to 2300 m in the Americas and possibly higher in Africa. Countries or areas where the yellow fever virus is present far exceed those officially reported. Some countries may have no reported cases simply because of a high level of vaccine coverage against yellow fever in the population or because of poor surveillance. A revision of the risk classification of countries and areas recommended for yellow fever vaccination is reflected in this year's edition (Country List and Annex 1).
Risk for travellers	Travellers are at risk in all countries or areas at risk of yellow fever transmission (Country List and Annex 1). Yellow fever vaccination is *generally not recommended* in areas where there is low potential for exposure to yellow fever virus. However, vaccination might be considered for a small subset of travellers to these areas, who are at increased risk of exposure to yellow fever virus (e.g. prolonged travel, extensive exposure to mosquitoes, inability to avoid mosquito bites). When considering vaccination, any traveller must take into account the risk of being infected with yellow fever virus, country entry requirements, as well as individual risk factors (e.g. age, immune status) for serious vaccine-associated adverse events.
Precautions	Avoid mosquito bites during the day and early evening (Chapter 3).
Vaccine	The 17D vaccine, which is based on a live, attenuated viral strain, is the only commercially available yellow fever vaccine. It is given as a single subcutaneous (or intramuscular) injection. Yellow fever vaccine is highly effective (approaching 100%). All individuals aged 9 months or older and living in countries or areas at risk should receive yellow fever vaccine.

Precautions and contraindications

The safety of the vaccine is considered to be excellent for the majority of travellers although some vaccine recipients develop mild reactions, including myalgia and headache. Contraindications include true allergy to egg protein, immunodeficiency (congenital or acquired) and symptomatic HIV infection (Chapter 9). There is a theoretical risk of harm to the fetus if the vaccine is given during pregnancy and vaccination of nursing mothers should be avoided because of the risk for the transmission of 17D virus to and encephalitis in the breast-fed infant. These risks must be weighed against the risk to the mother of remaining unvaccinated and travelling to an area where exposure to yellow fever virus may occur. In general, unvaccinated pregnant or nursing women should be advised not to travel to such areas.

Encephalitis has been reported as a rare event following vaccination, principally in infants under 6 months of age. As a result, the vaccine is contraindicated in infants under 6 months of age and is not recommended for those aged 6–8 months, except during epidemics when the risk of yellow fever transmission may be very high.

Vaccine-associated viscerotropic disease is a recently described adverse event that on very rare occasions has occurred after the first immunization with the yellow fever 17D vaccine. Onset is within 10 days of vaccination and the pathological process is characterized by severe multi-organ failure and an overall case–fatality rate in excess of 60%. Known risk factors include a history of thymus disease (e.g. thymoma or thymectomy) and aged 60 years and older.

Increased incidence of vaccine-associated neurotropic disease (e.g. meningoen-cephalitis, acute disseminated encephalomyelitis and Guillain–Barré syndrome) has been reported in infants under 6 months of age and individuals aged 60 years and older. The incidence rate reported in travellers from the United States and Europe ranges between 0.13 and 0.8 per 100 000 doses.

Yellow fever vaccination is required for travellers to certain countries and recommended for all travellers to countries or areas with risk of yellow fever transmission (Country list and Annex 1). The risk to unvaccinated individuals who visit countries or areas where there may be yellow fever transmission is often greater than the risk of a vaccine-related adverse event. While yellow fever vaccination should be encouraged as a key prevention strategy, it is important to screen travel itineraries and carefully evaluate the potential risk of systemic illness after yellow fever vaccination. Great care should be exercised not to prescribe yellow fever vaccination to individuals who are not at risk of exposure to infection, based on an accurate assessment of the travel itinerary. Although vaccination is generally not recommended for travellers going to areas where there is low potential for exposure to yellow fever virus. However, vaccination might be considered for a small subset of travellers to these areas, who are at increased risk of exposure to yellow fever virus (e.g. prolonged travel, extensive exposure to mosquitoes, inability to avoid mosquito bites). When considering vaccination, any traveller must take into account the risk of being infected with yellow fever virus, country entry requirements, as well as individual risk factors (e.g. age, immune status) for serious vaccine-associated adverse events.

Type of vaccine:	Live, attenuated
Number of doses:	One dose of 0.5 ml
Booster:	Currently every 10 years (if re-certification is needed)
Contraindications:	Infants aged less than 6 months; history of allergy to egg or to any of the vaccine components, or hypersensitivity to a previous dose of the vaccine; thymoma or history of thymectomy, immunodeficiency from medication, disease or symptomatic HIV infection.
Adverse reactions:	Rarely, neurological (encephalitis) or multi-organ failure resembling wild-type yellow fever
Before departure:	International certificate of vaccination becomes valid 10 days after vaccination.

Recommended for:	All travellers to countries and areas with risk of yellow fever transmission and when required by countries.
Special precautions:	Not recommended for infants aged 6–8 months, except during epidemics when the risk of YF virus transmission may be very high. Individuals aged 60 years and older are at increased risk for severe adverse events after vaccination. The risks and benefits of vaccination in this age group should be carefully considered before vaccination. The vaccine is not recommended during pregnancy or breastfeeding. However, pregnant or nursing women may be vaccinated during epidemics or if traveling to country or area at risk of transmission is unavoidable.

For the international certificate of vaccination, see below under "Required vaccinations".

Yellow fever vaccination recommendations in Africa, 2010

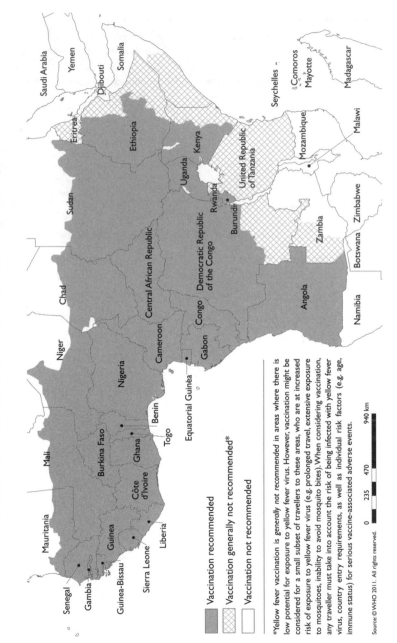

Vaccination recommended

Vaccination generally not recommended*

Vaccination not recommended

*Yellow fever vaccination is *generally not recommended* in areas where there is low potential for exposure to yellow fever virus. However, vaccination might be considered for a small subset of travellers to these areas, who are at increased risk of exposure to yellow fever virus (e.g. prolonged travel, extensive exposure to mosquitoes, inability to avoid mosquito bites). When considering vaccination, any traveller must take into account the risk of being infected with yellow fever virus, country entry requirements, as well as individual risk factors (e.g. age, immune status) for serious vaccine-associated adverse events.

0   235   470   940 km

Yellow fever vaccination recommendations in the Americas, 2010

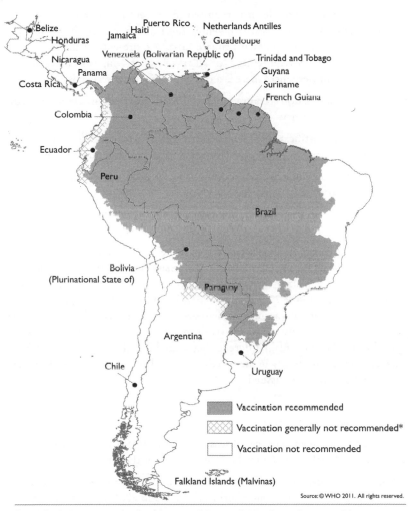

Belize
Honduras
Nicaragua
Panama
Costa Rica
Colombia
Ecuador
Peru
Bolivia
(Plurinational State of)
Chile
Argentina

Puerto Rico
Haiti
Jamaica
Venezuela (Bolivarian Republic of)

Netherlands Antilles
Guadeloupe
Trinidad and Tobago
Guyana
Suriname
French Guiana

Brazil

Paraguay

Uruguay

Falkland Islands (Malvinas)

Vaccination recommended

Vaccination generally not recommended*

Vaccination not recommended

*Yellow fever vaccination is *generally not recommended* in areas where there is low potential for exposure to yellow fever virus. However, vaccination might be considered for a small subset of travellers to these areas, who are at increased risk of exposure to yellow fever virus (e.g. prolonged travel, extensive exposure to mosquitoes, inability to avoid mosquito bites). When considering vaccination, any traveller must take into account the risk of being infected with yellow fever virus, country entry requirements, as well as individual risk factors (e.g. age, immune status) for serious vaccine-associated adverse events.

6.3 Required vaccinations

6.3.1 Yellow fever

Vaccination against yellow fever is required to prevent the importation of yellow fever virus into countries where yellow fever does not occur but where the mosquito vector and non-human primate hosts are present. In those settings, vaccination is an entry requirement for all travellers arriving (including airport transit) from countries where there is a risk of yellow fever transmission.

If yellow fever vaccination is contraindicated for medical reasons, a letter of medical exemption is necessary.

The international certificate of vaccination for yellow fever vaccine becomes valid 10 days after primary vaccination and remains valid for a period of 10 years.

For information on countries that require proof of yellow fever vaccination as a condition of entry, see Country list.

Travellers should be aware that the absence of a requirement for vaccination does not imply that there is no risk of exposure to yellow fever in the country.

Explanatory notes on the international certificate of vaccination are included at the end of this chapter. A revision of the International Health Regulations was adopted on 23 May 2005 by the World Health Assembly, and these Regulations entered into force in June 2007 (Annex 2). As from June 2007, the previous "International certificate of vaccination or revaccination against yellow fever" has been replaced by the "International certificate of vaccination or prophylaxis". It should be noted that the main difference between this and the previous certificate is the requirement to specify in the space provided that yellow fever is the disease for which the certificate is issued.

6.3.2 Meningococcal disease

Vaccination against meningococcal disease is required by Saudi Arabia for pilgrims visiting Mecca for the Hajj (annual pilgrimage) or for the Umrah.

Following the occurrence of cases of meningococcal disease associated with *Neisseria meningitidis* W-135 among pilgrims in 2000 and 2001, the current requirement is for vaccination with tetravalent vaccine (A, C, Y and W-135). Vaccine requirements for Hajj pilgrims are issued each year and published in the *Weekly Epidemiological Record.*

6.3.3 Poliomyelitis

Some polio-free countries may require travellers from countries or areas report-ing wild polio viruses (see http://www.polioeradication.org/Dataandmonitoring/Poliothisweek.aspx) to be immunized against polio in order to obtain an entry visa. Updates are published in the *Weekly Epidemiological Record*. For more information on Hajj visa requirements, Chapter 9.

6.4 Special groups

6.4.1 Infants and young children

Because not all vaccines can be administered to the very young, it is especially important to ensure protection against health hazards such as foodborne illnesses and mosquito bites by means other than vaccination.

Some vaccines can be administered at birth (BCG, oral poliomyelitis vaccine, hepatitis B); others, e.g. diphtheria/tetanus/pertussis, cannot be given before a certain age; Japanese encephalitis cannot be given before 6 months and yellow fever not before 9 months. Because it may be difficult to reduce children's exposure to environmental dangers, it is particularly important to ensure that their routine vaccinations are fully up to date. A child who travels abroad before completing the full schedule of routine vaccines is at risk from vaccine-preventable diseases.

6.4.2 Adolescents and young adults

Adolescents and young adults make up the largest group of travellers and the group most likely to acquire sexually transmitted diseases or other travel-related infections. They are particularly at risk when travelling on a limited budget and using accommodation of poor standard (e.g. when backpacking), or when their lifestyle includes risky sexual behaviour and other risks taken under the influ-ence of alcohol or drugs. Because risk reduction through behaviour modification may not be reliable, this age group should be strongly encouraged to accept all appropriate vaccines before travel and to adhere to other precautions for avoiding infectious diseases.

6.4.3 Frequent travellers

Individuals who travel widely, usually by air, often become lax about taking pre-cautions regarding their health. Having travelled numerous times without major health upsets, they may neglect to check that they are adequately vaccinated. Such travellers pose a special problem for health advisers who should, nonetheless, encourage compliance.

6.4.4 Pregnant women

Pregnancy should not deter a woman from receiving vaccines that are safe and will protect both her health and that of her unborn child. However, care must be taken to avoid the inappropriate administration of certain vaccines that could harm the unborn baby. Killed or inactivated vaccines such as influenza vaccine, toxoids and polysaccharides can generally be given during pregnancy, as can oral poliomyelitis vaccine. Live vaccines are generally contraindicated because of largely theoretical risks to the baby; measles, mumps, rubella, varicella and yellow fever vaccines should therefore be avoided in pregnancy. The risks and benefits should nevertheless be examined in each individual case. Vaccination against yellow fever may be considered in early pregnancy depending upon the risk (see Table 6.2). For more detailed information, see the specific vaccine position papers at: http://www.who.int/immunization/documents/positionpapers_intro/en/index.html

6.4.5 Elderly travellers

In general, vaccination of healthy elderly travellers does not differ from vaccination of younger adults. However, special considerations arise if the elderly traveller has not been fully immunized in the past and/or has existing medical problems.

Many elderly people may have never been vaccinated with the vaccines used in routine childhood immunization programmes or may have neglected to keep up the recommended schedule of booster doses. As a consequence, they may be susceptible to diseases such as diphtheria, tetanus and poliomyelitis as well as to other infections present at the travel destination.

Elderly travellers who have never been vaccinated should be offered a full primary course of vaccination against diphtheria, tetanus, poliomyelitis and hepatitis B. In addition, those who are not immune to hepatitis A should be vaccinated against this disease before travelling to a developing country.

Since the elderly are at risk for severe and complicated influenza, regular annual vaccination is recommended. For travellers from one hemisphere to the other, vaccine against the currently circulating strains of influenza is unlikely to be obtainable before arrival at the travel destination. Those arriving shortly before, or early during, the influenza season, and planning to stay for more than 2–3 weeks, should arrange vaccination as soon as possible after arrival. Pneumococcal poly-

Table 6.2 **Vaccination in pregnancy**

Vaccine	Use in pregnancy	Comments
BCG[a]	No	
Cholera	Yes, administer oral inactivated vaccine if indicated	
Hepatitis A	Yes, administer if indicated	
Hepatitis B	Yes, administer if indicated	
Influenza	Yes, administer if indicated	Use inactivated vaccine
Japanese encephalitis	No for live vaccine	Safety not determined
Measles[a]	No	
Meningococcal disease	Yes, administer if indicated	
Mumps[a]	No	
Poliomyelitis:		
OPV[a]	Yes, administer if indicated	
IPV	Yes, administer if indicated	
Rubella[a]	No	
Tetanus/diphtheria	Yes, administer if indicated	
Rabies	Yes, administer if indicated	
Typhoid Ty21a[a]		Safety not determined
Varicella[a]	No	
Yellow fever[a]	Yes, administer if indicated	Avoid unless at high risk

[a] Live vaccine.

saccharide vaccine may be considered for elderly travellers in view of the risk of pneumococcal pneumonia following influenza infection. On the other hand, this vaccine has not been demonstrated to prevent non-bacteraemic pneumonia among individuals at the highest risk of influenza-related morbidity and mortality.

Special considerations arise in the case of elderly travellers with pre-existing chronic health problems (see below).

6.4.6 Travellers with chronic medical problems

Travellers with chronic medical conditions involving impaired immunity, including cancer, diabetes mellitus, HIV infection and treatment with immunosuppressive drugs, may be at risk of severe complications following administration of vaccines that contain live organisms. Consequently, it may be advisable for these travellers to avoid measles, oral poliomyelitis, yellow fever, varicella and BCG vaccines. For travel to a country where yellow fever vaccination is required, a letter of medical exemption should be issued.

Travellers with chronic cardiovascular and/or respiratory conditions or diabetes mellitus are at high risk for severe influenza and its complications. Regular annual vaccination against influenza is recommended. For travel from one hemisphere to the other shortly before, or early, during the influenza season, vaccination should be sought as soon as possible after arrival at the travel destination.

For those who lack a functional spleen, additional vaccines are advised: Hib, meningococcal vaccine (conjugate C or quadrivalent conjugate vaccine) and possibly pneumococcal vaccination should be considered, in addition to regular vaccination against influenza.

6.4.7 HIV-positive travellers

Chapter 9.

6.5 Adverse reactions and contraindications
(see Tables 6.3 and 6.4)

6.5.1 Reactions to vaccines

While vaccines are generally both effective and safe, no vaccine is totally safe for all recipients. Vaccination may sometimes cause certain mild side-effects: local reaction, slight fever and other systemic symptoms may develop as part of the normal immune response. In addition, certain components of the vaccine (e.g. aluminium adjuvant, antibiotics or preservatives) occasionally cause reactions. A successful vaccine reduces these reactions to a minimum while inducing maximum immunity. Serious reactions are rare. Health workers who administer vaccines have an obligation to inform recipients of known adverse reactions and the likelihood of their occurrence.

A known contraindication should be clearly marked on a traveller's vaccination card, so that the vaccine may be avoided in future. In exceptional circumstances, the medical adviser may consider the risk of a particular disease to be greater than the theoretical risk of administering the vaccine and will advise vaccination.

6.5.2 Common mild vaccine reactions

Most vaccines produce some mild local and/or systemic reactions relatively frequently. These reactions generally occur within a day or two of immunization. However, the systemic symptoms that may arise with measles or MMR vaccine occur 5–12 days after vaccination. Fever and/or rash occur in 5–15% of measles/MMR vaccine recipients during this time, but only 3% are attributable to the vaccine; the rest may be classed as background events, i.e. normal events of childhood.

6.5.3 Uncommon, severe adverse reactions

Most of the rare vaccine reactions (detailed in Table 6.3) are self-limiting and do not lead to long-term problems. Anaphylaxis, for example, although potentially fatal, can be treated and has no long-term effects.

All serious reactions should be reported immediately to the relevant national health authority and marked on the vaccination card. In addition, the patient and relatives should be instructed to avoid the vaccination in the future.

6.5.4 Contraindications

The main contraindications to the administration of vaccines are summarized in Table 6.4.

Table 6.3 **Uncommon severe adverse reactions**

Vaccine	Possible adverse reaction	Expected rate[a] per million doses
BCG	Suppurative lymphadenitis	100–1000 (mostly in immunodeficient individuals)
	BCG-osteitis	1–700 (rarely with current vaccines)
	Disseminated BCG infection	0.19–1.56
Cholera	NR[b]	—
DTP	Persistent crying	1000–60 000
	Seizures	570
	Hypotonic–hyporesponsive episode	570
	Anaphylaxis	20
Haemophilus influenzae	NR	—

Vaccine	Possible adverse reaction	Expected rate[a] per million doses
Hepatitis A	NR	—
Hepatitis B[c]	Anaphylaxis	1–2
Influenza	Guillain–Barré syndrome	<1
Japanese encephalitis	Neurological event (mouse-brain only) Hypersensitivity	Rare 1800–6400
Measles	Febrile seizure Thrombocytopenic purpura Anaphylaxis Encephalitis	333 33–45 1–50 1 (unproven)
Meningococcal disease	Anaphylaxis	1
Mumps	Depends on strain – aseptic meningitis	0–500
Pneumococcal	Anaphylaxis	Very rare
Poliomyelitis (OPV)	Vaccine-associated paralytic poliomyelitis	1.4–3.4
Poliomyelitis (IPV)	NR	—
Rabies	Animal brain tissue only – neuroparalysis Cell-derived – allergic reactions	17–44 Rare
Rubella	Arthralgia/arthritis/arthropathy	None or very rare
Tetanus	Brachial neuritis Anaphylaxis	5–10 1–6
Tick-borne encephalitis	NR	—
Typhoid fever	Parenteral vaccine – various Oral vaccine – NR	Very rare —
Yellow fever	Encephalitis (<6 months) Allergy/anaphylaxis Viscerotropic disease	500–4000 5–20 0–4

[a] Precise rate may vary with survey method.

[b] NR = none reported.

[c] Although there have been anecdotal reports of demyelinating disease following hepatitis B vaccine, there is no scientific evidence for a causal relationship.

Table 6.4 **Contraindications to vaccines**

Vaccine	Contraindications
All	An anaphylactic reaction[a] following a previous dose of a particular vaccine is a true contraindication to further immunization with the antigen concerned and a subsequent dose should not be given. Current serious illness
MMR, BCG, JE, varicella	Pregnancy Severe immunodeficiency
Yellow fever	Severe egg allergy Severe immunodeficiency (from medication or disease or symptomatic) Pregnancy HIV infection[b]
BCG	HIV infection
Influenza	Severe egg allergy
Pertussis-containing vaccines	Anaphylactic reaction to a previous dose

[a] Generalized urticaria, difficulty in breathing, swelling of the mouth and throat, hypotension or shock.

[b] In many industrialized countries, yellow fever vaccine is administered to individuals who have symptomatic HIV infection or who are suffering from other immunodeficiency diseases, provided that their CD4 count is at least 200 cells/mm^3 and if they plan to visit countries or areas at risk.

Further reading

Global Influenza Surveillance Network (FluNet): http://www.who.int/GlobalAtlas/

Information on safety of vaccines from the Global Advisory Committee on Vaccine Safety: http://www.who.int/vaccine_safety/en/

WHO information on vaccine preventable diseases: http://www.who.int/immunization/en/

WHO vaccine position papers: http://www.who.int/immunization/documents/positionpapers_intro/en/index.html

International certificate of vaccination

A revision of the International Health Regulations, referred to as IHR (2005), was unanimously adopted on 23 May 2005 by the World Health Assembly, and these Regulations entered into force in June 2007 (Annex 2). As from 15 June 2007, the previous "International certificate of vaccination or revaccination against yellow fever" has been replaced by the "International certificate of vaccination or prophylaxis", as follows:

International certificate of vaccination or prophylaxis

Model international certificate of vaccination or prophylaxis

This is to certify that [name] ....

date of birth .... sex ....

nationality ....

national identification document, if applicable ....

whose signature follows ....

has on the date indicated been vaccinated or received prophylaxis against [name of disease or condition] ....
in accordance with the International Health Regulations.

Vaccine or pro- phylaxis	Date	Signature and professional status of supervising clinician	Manufacturer and batch no. of vaccine or prophylaxis	Certificate valid from .... until	Official stamp of administering centre
1.					
2.					

This certificate is valid only if the vaccine or prophylaxis used has been approved by the World Health Organization.[1]

This certificate must be signed in the hand of the clinician, who shall be a medical practitioner or other authorized health worker, supervising the administration of the vaccine or prophylaxis. The certificate must also bear the official stamp of the administering centre; however, this shall not be an accepted substitute for the signature.

Any amendment of this certificate, or erasure, or failure to complete any part of it, may render it invalid.

The validity of this certificate shall extend until the date indicated for the particular vaccination or prophylaxis. The certificate shall be fully completed in English or in French. The certificate may also be completed in another language on the same document, in addition to either English or French.

---

[1] See http://www.who.int/immunization_standards/vaccine_quality/pq_suppliers/en/index.html WHO Technical Report Series, No. 872, 1998, Annex 1 (http://www.who.int/biologicals). *Note*: since this list was issued, the following changes have taken place: Evans Medical is now Novartis Vaccines; Connaught Laboratories and Pasteur Merieux are now sanofi pasteur; Robert Koch Institute has ceased production.

CHAPTER 7

Malaria

7.1 Background

Malaria is a common and life-threatening disease in many tropical and subtropical areas. There are currently over 100 countries or areas at risk of malaria transmission, which are visited by more than 125 million international travellers every year.

Each year many international travellers fall ill with malaria while visiting countries or areas at risk, and well over 10 000 are reported to become ill after returning home; however, underreporting means that the real figure may be considerably higher. International travellers to countries or areas at risk of transmission arriving from countries or areas of no risk are at high risk of malaria and its consequences because they lack immunity. Immigrants from countries or areas at risk living in countries or areas of no risk and who return to their home countries to visit friends and relatives are similarly at risk because of waning or absent immunity. Fever occurring in a traveller within 3 months of leaving a country or area at risk of malaria is a medical emergency and should be investigated urgently.

Travellers who fall ill during travel may find it difficult to access reliable medical care. Travellers who develop malaria upon returning to a country or area of no risk present particular problems: doctors may be unfamiliar with malaria, the diagnosis may be delayed, and effective antimalarial medicines may not be registered and/or available, resulting in progression to severe and complicated malaria and, consequently, high case-fatality rates.

7.1.2 Cause

Malaria is caused by the protozoan parasite *Plasmodium*. Human malaria is caused by four different species of *Plasmodium*: *P. falciparum*, *P. malariae*, *P. ovale* and *P. vivax*.

Humans occasionally become infected with *Plasmodium* species that normally infect animals, such as *P. knowlesi*. As yet, there are no reports of human-mosquito-human transmission of such "zoonotic" forms of malaria.

7.1.3 Transmission

The malaria parasite is transmitted by female *Anopheles* mosquitoes, which bite mainly between dusk and dawn.

7.1.4 Nature of the disease

Malaria is an acute febrile illness with an incubation period of 7 days or longer. Thus, a febrile illness developing less than 1 week after the first possible exposure is not malaria.

The most severe form is caused by *P. falciparum*; variable clinical features include fever, chills, headache, muscular aching and weakness, vomiting, cough, diarrhoea and abdominal pain. Other symptoms related to organ failure may supervene, such as acute renal failure, pulmonary oedema, generalized convulsions, circulatory collapse, followed by coma and death. The initial symptoms, which may be mild, may not be easy to recognize as being due to malaria.

It is important that the possibility of falciparum malaria is considered in all cases of unexplained fever starting at any time between 7 days after the first possible exposure to malaria and 3 months (or, rarely, later) after the last possible exposure. Any individual who experiences a fever in this interval should immediately seek diagnosis and effective treatment, and inform medical personnel of the possible exposure to malaria infection. Falciparum malaria may be fatal if treatment is delayed beyond 24 h after the onset of clinical symptoms.

Young children, pregnant women, people who are immunosuppressed and elderly travellers are particularly at risk of severe disease. Malaria, particularly *P. falciparum*, in non-immune pregnant travellers increases the risk of maternal death, miscarriage, stillbirth and neonatal death.

The forms of human malaria caused by other *Plasmodium* species cause significant morbidity but are rarely life-threatening. Cases of severe *P. vivax* malaria have recently been reported among populations living in (sub)tropical countries or areas at risk. *P. vivax* and *P. ovale* can remain dormant in the liver. Relapses caused by these persistent liver forms ("hypnozoites") may appear months, and rarely several years, after exposure. Relapses are not prevented by current chemoprophylactic regimens, with the exception of primaquine. Latent blood infection with *P. malariae* may be present for many years, but it is very rarely life-threatening.

In recent years, sporadic cases of travellers' malaria due to *P. knowlesi* have been reported. Humans can be infected with this "monkey malaria" parasite while staying in rainforests and/or their fringe areas in south-east Asia, within the range of the natural monkey hosts and mosquito vector of this infection. These areas include parts of Cambodia, China, Indonesia, Laos, Malaysia, Myanmar, the Philippines, Singapore, Thailand and Viet Nam. The parasite has a life-cycle of 24 h and can give rise to daily fever spikes occurring 9–12 days after infection. Symptoms may be atypical. Severe *P. knowlesi* malaria with organ failure may occur, and sporadic fatal outcomes have been described. *P. knowlesi* has no persistent liver forms and relapses do not occur. Travellers to forested areas of south-east Asia where human *P. knowlesi* infections have been reported should protect themselves against mosquito bites between dusk and dawn to prevent infection and take the usual chemoprophylaxis where indicated (see Country list).

7.1.5 Geographical distribution

The current distribution of malaria in the world is shown on the map in this chapter; affected countries and territories are listed both at the end of this chapter and in the Country list. The risk for travellers of contracting malaria is highly variable from country to country and even between areas in a country, and this must be considered in any discussion of appropriate preventive measures.

In many countries or area at risk, the main urban areas – but not necessarily the outskirts of towns – are free of malaria transmission. However, malaria can occur in the main urban areas of Africa and, to a lesser extent, India. There is usually less risk at altitudes above 1500 m, although in favourable climatic conditions the disease can occur at altitudes up to almost 3000 m. The risk of infection may also vary according to the season, being highest at the end of the rainy season or soon after.

There is no risk of malaria in many tourist destinations in south-east Asia, the Caribbean and Latin America.

7.1.6   Risk for travellers

During the transmission season in countries or areas at risk, all non-immune travellers exposed to mosquito bites, especially between dusk and dawn, are at risk of malaria. This includes previously semi-immune travellers who have lost or partially lost their immunity during stays of 6 months or more in countries or areas of no risk. Children who have migrated to countries and areas of no risk are particularly at risk when they travel to malarious areas to visit friends and relatives.

Most cases of falciparum malaria in travellers occur because of poor adherence to, or complete failure to use medicines, or use of inappropriate prophylactic malaria

Malaria, countries or areas at risk of transmission, 20010

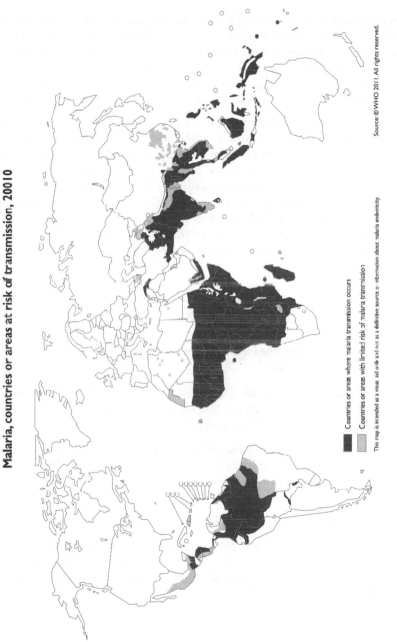

Countries or areas where malaria transmission occurs

Countries or areas with limited risk of malaria transmission

drug regimens, combined with failure to take adequate precautions against mosquito bites. Studies on travellers' behaviour have shown that adherence to treatment can be improved if travellers are informed of the risk of infection and believe in the benefit of prevention strategies. Late-onset vivax and ovale malaria may occur despite effective prophylaxis, as they cannot be prevented with currently recommended prophylactic regimens which act only against blood-stage parasites.

Malaria risk is not evenly distributed where the disease is prevalent. Travellers to countries where the degree of malaria transmission varies in different areas should seek advice on the risk in the particular zones that they will be visiting. If specific information is not available before travelling, it is recommended that precautions appropriate for the highest reported risk for the area or country should be taken; these precautions can be adjusted when more information becomes available on arrival. This applies particularly to individuals backpacking to remote places and visiting areas where diagnostic facilities and medical care are not readily available. Travellers staying overnight in rural areas may be at highest risk.

7.2 Precautions

Travellers and their advisers should note the four principles – the ABCD – of malaria protection:

- Be **A**ware of the risk, the incubation period, the possibility of delayed onset, and the main symptoms.
- Avoid being **B**itten by mosquitoes, especially between dusk and dawn.
- Take antimalarial drugs (**C**hemoprophylaxis) when appropriate, to prevent infection from developing into clinical disease.
- Immediately seek **D**iagnosis and treatment if a fever develops 1 week or more after entering an area where there is a malaria risk and up to 3 months (or, rarely, later) after departure from a risk area.

7.2.1 Protection against mosquito bites

All travellers should be advised that individual protection from mosquito bites between dusk and dawn is their first line of defence against malaria. Practical measures for protection are described in Chapter 3, in the section "Protection against vectors".

7.2.2 Chemoprophylaxis

The most appropriate chemoprophylactic antimalarial drug(s) (if any) for the destination(s) should be prescribed in the correct dosages (see Country list and Table 7.2).

Travellers and their doctors should be aware that **no antimalarial prophylactic regimen gives complete protection,** but good chemoprophylaxis (adherence to the recommended drug regimen) significantly reduces the risk of fatal disease. The following should also be taken into account:

● Dosing schedules for children should be based on body weight.

● Antimalarials that have to be taken daily should be started the day before arrival in the risk area (or earlier if drug tolerability needs to be checked before departure).

● Weekly chloroquine should be started 1 week before arrival.

● Weekly mefloquine should preferably be started 2–3 weeks before departure, to achieve higher pre-travel blood levels and to allow side-effects to be detected before travel so that possible alternatives can be considered.

● All prophylactic drugs should be taken with unfailing regularity for the duration of the stay in the malaria risk area, and should be continued for 4 weeks after the last possible exposure to infection, since parasites may still emerge from the liver during this period. The single exception is atovaquone–proguanil, which can be stopped 1 week after return because of its effect on early liver-stage parasites (liver schizonts). However, in case daily doses are skipped while the traveller is exposed to malaria risk, atovaquone–proguanil prophylaxis should also be taken for 4 weeks after return.

● Depending on the type of malaria at the destination, travellers should be advised about possible late-onset *P. ovale* and *P. vivax.*

Depending on the type of malaria risk in the country or area visited (see Country list), the recommended prevention method may be mosquito bite prevention only, or mosquito bite prevention in combination with chemoprophylaxis or stand-by emergency treatment, as follows (see also Table 7.2 for details of individual drugs)

	Malaria risk	Type of prevention
Type I	Very limited risk of malaria transmission	Mosquito bite prevention only
Type II	Risk of *P. vivax* malaria only; or fully chloroquine-sensitive *P. falciparum*	Mosquito bite prevention plus chloroquine chemoprophylaxis
Type III[a]	Risk of *P. vivax* and *P. falciparum* malaria transmission, combined with emerging chloroquine resistance	Mosquito bite prevention plus chloroquine+proguanil chemoprophylaxis
Type IV	(1) High risk of *P. falciparum* malaria, in combination with reported antimalarial drug resistance; or (2) Moderate/low risk of *P. falciparum* malaria, in combination with reported high levels of drug resistance[b]	Mosquito bite prevention plus atovaquone–proguanil, doxycycline or mefloquine chemoprophylaxis (select according to reported resistance pattern)

[a] The areas where Type III prevention is still an option are limited to Nepal, Sri Lanka and Tajikistan, and parts of Colombia and India. Type IV prevention can be used instead.

[b] Alternatively, when travelling to rural areas with multidrug-resistant malaria and only a very low risk of *P. falciparum* infection, mosquito bite prevention can be combined with stand-by emergency treatment (SBET).

There are specific contraindications and possible side-effects for all antimalarial drugs. Adverse reactions attributed to malaria chemoprophylaxis are common, but most are minor and do not affect the activities of the traveller. Serious adverse events – defined as constituting an apparent threat to life, requiring or prolonging hospitalization, or resulting in persistent or significant disability or incapacity – are rare and normally identified in postmarketing surveillance once a drug has been in use for some time. Severe neuropsychiatric disturbances (seizures, psychosis, encephalopathy) occur in approximately 1 in 10 000 travellers receiving mefloquine prophylaxis, and have also been reported for chloroquine at a similar rate. The risk of drug-associated adverse events should be weighed against the risk of malaria, especially *P. falciparum* malaria, and local drug-resistance patterns.

Each of the antimalarial drugs is contraindicated in certain groups and individuals, and the contraindications should be carefully observed (see Table 7.2) to reduce the risk of serious adverse reactions. Pregnant women, people travelling with young children, and people with chronic illnesses should seek individual medical advice. Any traveller who develops severe adverse-effects while using an anti-malarial should stop taking the drug and seek immediate medical attention. This applies particularly to neurological or psychological disturbances experienced with mefloquine prophylaxis. Mild nausea, occasional vomiting or loose stools should not prompt discontinuation of prophylaxis, but medical advice should be sought if symptoms persist.

Long-term chemoprophylaxis
Adherence and tolerability are important aspects of chemoprophylaxis in long-term travellers. There are few studies on chemoprophylaxis use during travel lasting more than 6 months.

- The risk of serious side-effects associated with long-term prophylactic use of chloroquine and proguanil is low, but retinal toxicity is of concern when a cumulative dose of 100 g of chloroquine is reached. Anyone who has taken 300 mg of chloroquine weekly for more than 5 years and requires further prophylaxis should be screened twice-yearly for early retinal changes. If daily doses of 100 mg chloroquine have been taken, screening should start after 3 years.

- Data indicate no increased risk of serious side-effects with long-term use of mefloquine if the drug is tolerated in the short term. Pharmacokinetic data indicate that mefloquine does not accumulate during long-term intake.

- Available data on long-term chemoprophylaxis with doxycycline (i.e. more than 12 months) are limited but reassuring. There are few data on long-term use of doxycycline in women, but use of this drug is associated with an increased frequency of vaginitis due to *Candida*.

- Atovaquone–proguanil is registered in European countries with a restriction on duration of use (varying from 5 weeks to 1 year); such restrictions do not apply in the United States.

7.3 Treatment

Early diagnosis and appropriate treatment can be life-saving. A blood sample should be taken from all travellers with suspected malaria and examined without delay for malaria parasites in an experienced, reliable laboratory. If no parasites are found in the first blood film, a series of blood samples should be taken at 6–12-h intervals and examined very carefully. Malaria rapid diagnostic tests can be useful in centres where malaria microscopy is unavailable. When laboratory analysis is delayed, physicians should begin treatment if the clinical indicators and travel history suggest malaria.

For travellers who are treated for malaria in countries or areas of no risk, the following principles apply:

- Patients are at high risk of malaria and its consequences because they are non-immune.

- If the patient has taken prophylaxis, the same medicine should not be used for treatment.

- Be alert to the possibility of mixed *P. falciparum–P. vivax* infections.

The following combination therapies are suitable for treatment of **uncomplicated falciparum malaria** in travellers on return in countries or areas of no risk:

- artemether–lumefantrine
- atovaquone–proguanil
- dihydroartemisinin–piperaquine
- quinine plus doxycycline or clindamycin.

The treatment for **vivax malaria** in travellers is as follows:

- Chloroquine combined with primaquine is the treatment of choice to achieve radical cure (i.e. to cure both the blood stage and liver stage infections, and thereby prevent both recrudescence and relapse).

- Dihydroartemisinin–piperaquine or artemether–lumefantrine should be given for chloroquine-resistant vivax malaria. Where these are not available, quinine can be used instead. They should be combined with primaquine.

- Travellers must be tested for glucose-6-phosphate dehydrogenase (G6PD) deficiency before receiving primaquine anti-relapse treatment. In moderate G6PD deficiency, primaquine should be given in an adjusted regimen of 0.75 mg base/kg body weight once a week for 8 weeks under medical observation for haemolysis. If significant haemolysis occurs on treatment, then primaquine should be stopped. In severe G6PD deficiency, primaquine should not be given.

- In mixed *P. falciparum/P. vivax* infections, the treatment for *P. falciparum* will usually also cure the attack of *P. vivax*, but primaquine should be added to achieve radical cure and prevent relapses.

Chemoprophylaxis and treatment of falciparum malaria are becoming more complex because *P. falciparum* is increasingly resistant to various antimalarial drugs. Chloroquine resistance of *P. vivax* is rare but increasing. Focal chloroquine resistance or prophylactic and/or treatment failure has since also been observed in

Afghanistan, Brazil, Cambodia, Colombia, Ethiopia, Guyana, India, Indonesia, Madagascar, Malaysia (Borneo), Myanmar, Pakistan, Papua New Guinea, Peru, the Republic of Korea, Solomon Islands, Sri Lanka, Thailand, Turkey, Vanuatu and Viet Nam. Chloroquine-resistant *P. malariae* has been reported from Indonesia.

Relapsing malaria caused by *P. ovale* can be treated with chloroquine and primaquine. **Malaria caused by *P. malariae*** can be treated with the standard regimen of chloroquine as for vivax malaria, but it does not require radical cure with primaquine because no hypnozoites are formed in infection with this species.

Returning travellers with **severe falciparum malaria** should be managed in an intensive care unit. Parenteral antimalarial treatment should be with artesunate (first choice), artemether or quinine. If these medicines are not available, parenteral quinidine should be used, with careful clinical and electrocardiographic monitoring.

On microscopy examination, the mature forms of *P. knowlesi* may be mistaken for *P. malariae*, while its ring forms may resemble *P. falciparum*. Knowlesi malaria can be treated with a standard regimen of chloroquine or with the antimalarials recommended for uncomplicated falciparum malaria. The clinical condition of patients infected with *P. knowlesi* may deteriorate quickly. Severe *P. knowlesi* malaria with organ failure may occur; it should be treated as for severe falciparum malaria.

P. knowlesi infection should always be considered in patients with a microscopy diagnosis of *P. malariae* and a travel history to forested areas of south-east Asia, including areas where malaria is not normally present.

The dosage regimens for the treatment of uncomplicated malaria are given in Table 7.3. Details of the clinical management of severe malaria are addressed in other WHO publications (see "Further reading" at the end of this chapter).

7.3.1 Treatment abroad

An individual who experiences a fever 1 week or more after entering an area of malaria risk should consult a physician or qualified malaria laboratory immediately to obtain a correct diagnosis and safe and effective treatment. In principle, travellers can be treated with artemisinin-based combination therapy (ACT) according to the national policy in the country they are visiting. National antimalarial drug policies for all countries and areas at risk are listed at http://www.who.int/malaria/treatmentpolicies.html.

In light of the spread of counterfeit drugs in some resource-poor settings, travellers may prefer to buy a reliable supply of a reserve antimalarial treatment before departure, so that they can be confident of drug quality should they become ill.

7.3.2 Stand-by emergency treatment

Many travellers will be able to obtain proper medical attention within 24 h of the onset of fever. For others, however, this may be impossible, particularly if they will be staying in remote locations. In such cases, travellers can be advised to carry anti-malarial drugs for self-administration ("stand-by emergency treatment - SBTE").

SBET may also be indicated for travellers in some occupational groups who make frequent short stops in countries or areas at risk over a prolonged period of time. Such travellers may choose to reserve chemoprophylaxis for high-risk areas and seasons only. However, they should continue to take measures to protect against mosquito bites and be prepared for an attack of malaria: they should always carry a course of antimalarial drugs for SBET, seek immediate medical care in case of fever, and take SBET if prompt medical help is not available.

Furthermore, SBET – combined with protection against mosquito bites – may be indicated for those who travel for 1 week or more to remote rural areas where there is multidrug-resistant malaria but a very low risk of infection, and the risk of side-effects of prophylaxis may outweigh that of contracting malaria. This may be the case in certain border areas of Thailand, Viet Nam and neighbouring countries in south-east Asia as well as parts of the Amazon basin.

Studies on the use of rapid diagnostic tests ("RDTs") have shown that untrained travellers experience major problems in the performance and interpretation of these tests, with an unacceptably high number of false-negative results. In addition, RDTs can be degraded by extremes of heat and humidity, becoming less sensitive.

Successful SBET depends crucially on travellers' behaviour, and health advisers need to spend time explaining the strategy. Travellers provided with SBET should be given clear and precise written instructions on the recognition of symptoms, when and how to take the treatment, possible side-effects, and the possibility of drug failure. If several people travel together, the individual dosages for SBET should be specified. Weight-based dosages for children need to be clearly indicated. **Travellers should realize that self-treatment is a first-aid measure and that they should still seek medical advice as soon as possible.**

In general, travellers carrying SBET should observe the following guidelines:

- Consult a physician immediately if fever occurs 1 week or more after entering an area with malaria risk.

- If it is impossible to consult a physician and/or establish a diagnosis within 24 h of the onset of fever, start the SBET and seek medical care as soon as possible for complete evaluation and to exclude other serious causes of fever.

- Do not treat suspected malaria with the same drugs as were used for prophylaxis.

- Vomiting of antimalarial drugs is less likely if fever is first lowered with antipyretics. A second full dose should be taken if vomiting occurs within 30 min of taking the drug. If vomiting occurs 30–60 min after a dose, an additional half-dose should be taken. Vomiting with diarrhoea may lead to treatment failure because of poor drug absorption.

- Complete the SBET course and resume antimalarial prophylaxis 1 week after the *first* treatment dose.

- The drug options for SBET are in principle the same as for treatment of uncomplicated malaria (Section 7.3). The choice will depend on the type of malaria in the area visited and the chemoprophylaxis regimen taken. Artemether–lumefantrine has been registered (in Switzerland and the United Kingdom) for use as SBET for travellers. Quinine is less feasible for SBET because of the long and cumbersome treatment regimen and the dose-dependent side-effects. If quinine is taken for SBET, at least 12 h should elapse between the *last* treatment dose of quinine and resumption of mefloquine prophylaxis to reduce the risk of drug interactions. Table 7.3 provides details on individual drugs.

7.3.3 Multidrug-resistant malaria

Multidrug-resistant malaria has been reported from south-east Asia (Cambodia, Myanmar, Thailand, Viet Nam) and the Amazon basin of South America, where it occurs in parts of Brazil, French Guiana and Suriname.

In border areas between Cambodia, Myanmar and Thailand, *P. falciparum* infections do not respond to treatment with chloroquine or sulfadoxine–pyrimethamine, sensitivity to quinine is reduced, treatment failures in excess of 50% with mefloquine are being reported, and – in south-western provinces of Cambodia on the border with Thailand – resistance to artesunate has emerged. In these situations, malaria prevention consists of personal protection measures in combination with atovaquone–proguanil or doxycycline as chemoprophylaxis. SBET with atovaquone–proguanil can be used in situations where the risk of infection is very low. However, these drugs cannot be given to pregnant women and young children. Since there is no prophylactic or SBET regimen that is both effective and safe for these groups in areas of multidrug-resistant malaria, pregnant women and young children should avoid travelling to these malarious areas. The emergence of artemisinin resistance on the Cambodia–Thailand border has implications for the management of malaria in international travellers for the following parts of south-east Asia: western Cambodia, eastern Myanmar and the Binc Phuc province of Viet Nam. To reduce the danger of introducing drug-resistant parasites to other endemic parts of the world, all malaria patients who have travelled in these areas should be promptly diagnosed and treated effectively. The addition of a single oral dose of primaquine (0.75 mg base/kg body weight, with 45 mg base maximum for adults) to treatment will accelerate the removal of gametocytes.

7.4 Special groups

Some groups of travellers, especially young children, pregnant women and immunosuppressed individuals, are at particular risk of serious consequences if they become infected with malaria. Recommendations for these groups are difficult to formulate because safety data are limited. The special concerns for immigrants from countries or areas at risk who live in countries or areas of no risk and return to their home countries to visit friends and relatives are addressed in Chapter 9.

7.4.1 Pregnant women

Malaria in a pregnant woman increases the risk of maternal death, miscarriage, stillbirth and low birth weight with associated risk of neonatal death.

Pregnant women should be advised to avoid travelling to areas where malaria transmission occurs. When travel cannot be avoided, it is very important to take effective preventive measures against malaria, even when travelling to areas where there is transmission only of vivax malaria. Pregnant women should seek medical help immediately if malaria is suspected; if this is not possible, they should take SBET. Medical help must be sought as soon as possible after starting SBET. There is very limited information on the safety and efficacy of most antimalarials in pregnancy, particularly during the first trimester. However, inadvertent exposure to antimalarials is **not** an indication for termination of the pregnancy.

Mosquito bite prevention
Pregnant women are particularly susceptible to mosquito bites and should therefore be vigilant in using protective measures, including insect repellents and insecticide-treated mosquito nets. They should take care not to exceed the recommended usage of insect repellents.

Chemoprophylaxis
In Type II areas, with exclusively *P. vivax* transmission or where *P. falciparum* can be expected to be fully sensitive to chloroquine, prophylaxis with chloroquine alone

may be used. In the few remaining Type III areas, prophylaxis with chloroquine plus proguanil can be safely prescribed, including during the first 3 months of pregnancy. In Type IV areas, mefloquine prophylaxis may be given during the second and third trimesters, but there is limited information on the safety of mefloquine during the first trimester. In light of the danger of malaria to mother and fetus, experts increasingly agree **that travel to a chloroquine-resistant *P. falciparum* area during the first trimester of pregnancy should be avoided or delayed at all costs; if this is truly impossible, good preventive measures should be taken, including prophylaxis with mefloquine where this is indicated.** Doxycycline is contraindicated during pregnancy. The atovaquone–proguanil combination has not been sufficiently investigated to be prescribed in pregnancy.

Treatment

Clindamycin and quinine are considered safe, including during the first trimester of pregnancy; artemisinin derivatives can be used to treat uncomplicated malaria in the second and third trimesters, and in the first trimester only if no other adequate medicines are available. Chloroquine can be safely used for treatment of vivax malaria in pregnancy, but primaquine anti-relapse treatment should be postponed until after delivery. Artemether–lumefantrine, atovaquone–proguanil and dihydroartemisinin–piperaquine have not been sufficiently investigated to be prescribed in pregnancy.

The recommended treatment for **uncomplicated falciparum malaria in the first trimester** is quinine +/– clindamycin. For the **second and third trimesters**, the options are: ACT in accordance with national policy; artesunate + clindamycin; or quinine + clindamycin.

Pregnant women with falciparum malaria, particularly in the second and third trimesters of pregnancy, are more likely than other adults to develop severe malaria, often complicated by hypoglycaemia and pulmonary oedema. Maternal mortality in severe malaria is approximately 50%, which is higher than in non-pregnant adults. Fetal death and premature labour are common. **Pregnant women with severe malaria** must be treated without delay with full doses of parenteral antimalarial treatment. In the **first trimester**, either quinine or artesunate can be used. In the **second and third trimesters**, artesunate is the first option and artemether the second option. Treatment must not be delayed: if only one of the drugs artesunate, artemether or quinine is available, it should be started immediately.

Information on the safety of antimalarial drugs during breastfeeding is provided in Tables 7.2 and 7.3.

7.4.2 Women who may become pregnant during or after travel

Malaria prophylaxis may be taken, but pregnancy should preferably be avoided during the period of drug intake and for 1 week after doxycycline, 3 weeks after atovaquone–proguanil, and 3 months after the last dose of mefloquine prophylaxis. If pregnancy occurs during antimalarial prophylaxis, this is not considered to be an indication for pregnancy termination.

7.4.3 Young children

Falciparum malaria in a young child is a medical emergency. It may be rapidly fatal. Early symptoms are atypical and difficult to recognize, and life-threatening complications can occur within hours of the initial symptoms. Medical help should be sought immediately if a child develops a febrile illness within 3 months (or, rarely, later) of travelling to a country or area at risk. Laboratory confirmation of diagnosis should be requested immediately, and treatment with an effective anti-malarial drug initiated as soon as possible. In infants, malaria should be suspected even in non-febrile illness.

Parents should be advised not to take infants or young children to areas where there is risk of falciparum malaria. If travel cannot be avoided, children must be very carefully protected against mosquito bites and be given appropriate chemo-prophylactic drugs. Long-term travellers and expatriates should adjust the chemo-prophylaxis dosage according to the increasing weight of the growing child.

Mosquito bite prevention

Infants should be kept under insecticide-treated mosquito nets as much as possible between dusk and dawn. The manufacturer's instructions on the use of insect repellents should be followed diligently, and the recommended usage must not be exceeded.

Chemoprophylaxis

Chloroquine, proguanil and mefloquine are considered compatible with breastfeed-ing. Breastfed, as well as bottle-fed, infants should be given chemoprophylaxis since they are not protected by the mother's prophylaxis. Dosage schedules for children should be based on body weight, and tablets should be crushed and ground as necessary. The bitter taste of the tablets can be disguised with jam or other foods. Chloroquine and proguanil are safe for infants and young children but their use is now very limited because of spreading chloroquine resistance. Mefloquine may be given to infants of more than 5 kg body weight. Atovaquone–proguanil is generally not recommended for prophylaxis in children who weigh less than 11 kg, because of limited data; in Belgium, Canada, France and the United States it is given for prophylaxis in infants of more than 5 kg body weight. Doxycycline is contraindicated in children below 8 years of age. All antimalarial drugs should be kept out of the reach of children and stored in childproof containers; chloroquine is particularly toxic in case of overdose.

Treatment

Acutely ill children with falciparum malaria require careful clinical monitoring as their condition may deteriorate rapidly. Every effort should be made to give oral treatment and ensure that it is retained. ACT as per national policy may be used as first-line treatment while abroad. Oral treatment options for SBET and returning travellers are: artemether–lumefantrine (not recommended under 5 kg because of lack of data), atovaquone–proguanil (apparently safe in children weighing 5 kg or more, but data are limited), dihydroartemisinin–piperaquine (apparently safe in children weighing 10 kg or more, but data are limited) and quinine plus clindamycin (safe, but data on clindamycin are limited). Quinine plus doxycycline is an option for children of 8 years and older. Parenteral treatment and admission to hospital are indicated for young children who cannot swallow antimalarials reliably.

Chloroquine can be safely given to treat *P. malariae*, *P. ovale* or *P. vivax* infections in young children. The lower age limit for anti-relapse treatment with primaquine has not been established; it is generally contraindicated in young infants.

Information on the safety of drugs for prophylaxis and treatment of young children is provided in Tables 7.2 and 7.3.

7.4.4 Immunosuppressed travellers

Immunosuppressed travellers are at increased risk of malaria disease, and prevention of malaria through avoidance of mosquito bites and use of chemoprophylaxis is particularly important. Individual pre-travel advice should be carefully sought. There may be an increased risk of antimalarial treatment failure in people living with HIV/AIDS. At present, however, there is insufficient information to permit modifications to treatment regimens to be recommended (Chapter 9).

Table 7.2 **Use of antimalarial drugs for prophylaxis in travellers**

| Generic name | Dosage regimen | Duration of prophylaxis | Use in special groups | | | Main contraindications[a] | Comments[a] |
			Pregnancy	Breast-feeding	Children		
Atovaquone–proguanil combination tablet	One dose daily. *11–20 kg*: 62.5 mg atovaquone plus 25 mg proguanil (1 paediatric tablet) daily *21–30 kg*: 2 paediatric tablets daily *31–40 kg*: 3 paediatric tablets daily *>40 kg*: 1 adult tablet (250 mg atovaquone plus 100 mg proguanil) daily	Start 1 day before departure and continue for 7 days after return	No data, not recommended	No data, not recommended	Not recommended <11 kg because of limited data	Hypersensitivity to atovaquone and/or proguanil; severe renal insufficiency (creatinine clearance <30 ml/min)	Take with food or milky drink to increase absorption. Registered in European countries for chemoprophylactic use with a restriction on duration of use (varying from 5 weeks to 1 year). Plasma concentrations of atovaquone are reduced when it is co-administered with rifampicin, rifabutin, metoclopramide or tetracycline. May interfere with live typhoid vaccine.
Chloroquine	5 mg base/kg weekly in one dose, or 10 mg base/kg weekly divided in 6 daily doses *Adult dose*: 300 mg chloroquine base weekly in one dose, or 600 mg chloroquine base weekly divided over 6 daily doses of 100 mg base (with one drug-free day per week)	Start 1 week before departure and continue for 4 weeks after return. If daily doses: start 1 day before departure	Safe	Safe	Safe	Hypersensitivity to chloroquine; history of epilepsy; psoriasis	Concurrent use of chloroquine may reduce the antibody response to intradermally administered human diploid-cell rabies vaccine.
Chloroquine–proguanil combination tablet	*>50 kg*: 100 mg chloroquine base plus 200 mg proguanil (1 tablet) daily	Start 1 day before departure and continue for 4 weeks after return	Safe	Safe	Tablet size not suitable for persons of <50 kg body weight	Hypersensitivity to chloroquine and/or proguanil; liver or kidney insufficiency; history of epilepsy; psoriasis	Concurrent use of chloroquine may reduce the antibody response to intradermally administered human diploid-cell rabies vaccine. May interfere with live typhoid vaccine.

[a] See package insert for full information on contraindications and precautions.

Table 7.2 Use of antimalarial drugs for prophylaxis in travellers *(continued)*

Generic name	Dosage regimen	Duration of prophylaxis	Use in special groups			Main contraindications[a]	Comments[a]
			Pregnancy	Breast-feeding	Children		
Doxycycline	1.5 mg salt/kg daily *Adult dose:* 1 tablet of 100 mg daily	Start 1 day before departure and continue for 4 weeks after return	Contra-indicated	Contra-indicated	Contra-indicated under 8 years of age	Hypersensitivity to tetra-cyclines; liver dysfunction	Doxycycline makes the skin more susceptible to sunburn. People with sensitive skin should use a highly protective (UVA) sunscreen and avoid prolonged direct sunlight, or switch to another drug. Doxycycline should be taken with plenty of water to prevent oesophageal irritation. Doxycycline may increase the risk of vaginal *Candida* infections. Studies indicate that the monohydrate form of the drug is better tolerated than the hyclate.
Mefloquine	5 mg/kg weekly *Adult dose:* 1 tablet of 250 mg weekly	Start at least 1 week (preferably 2–3 weeks) before departure and continue for 4 weeks after return	Not recommended in first trimester because of lack of data (also see pp. 156–159)	Safe	Not recommended under 5 kg because of lack of data	Hypersensitivity to mefloquine; psychiatric (including depression) or convulsive disorders; history of severe neuropsychiatric disease; concomitant halofantrine treatment; treatment with mefloquine in previous 4 weeks	Do not give mefloquine within 12 h of quinine treatment. Mefloquine and other cardioactive drugs may be given concomitantly only under close medical supervision. Ampicillin, tetracycline and metoclopramide may increase mefloquine blood levels. Do not give concomitantly with oral typhoid vaccine (see pp. 156–159).
Proguanil	3 mg/kg daily *Adult dose:* 2 tablets of 100 mg daily	Start 1 day before departure and continue for 4 weeks after return	Safe	Safe	Safe	Liver or kidney dysfunction	Use only in combination with chloroquine. Proguanil may interfere with live typhoid vaccine.

[a] See package insert for full information on contraindications and precautions.

Table 7.3 **Use of antimalarial drugs for treatment of uncomplicated malaria in travellers**

| Generic name | Dosage regimen | Use in special groups | | | Main contraindications[a] | Comments[a] |
		Pregnancy	Breast-feeding	Children		
Artemether–lumefantrine combination tablet	3-day course of 6 doses total, taken at 0, 8, 24, 36, 48 and 60 h *5–14 kg*: 1 tablet (20 mg artemether plus 120 mg lumefantrine) per dose *15–24 kg*: 2 tablets per dose *25–34 kg*: 3 tablets per dose *≥35 kg*: 4 tablets per dose	No data, not recommended	No data, not recommended	Not recommended under 5 kg because of lack of data	Hypersensitivity to artemether and/or lumefantrine	Must be taken with fatty foods to improve absorption. A flavoured dispersible paediatric formulation is now available, enhancing its use in young children.
Atovaquone–proguanil combination tablet	One dose daily for 3 consecutive days *5–8 kg*: 2 paediatric tablets daily (at 62.5 mg atovaquone plus 25 mg proguanil per tablet) *9–10 kg*: 3 paediatric tablets daily *11–20 kg*: 1 adult tablet (250 mg atovaquone plus 100 mg proguanil) daily *21–30 kg*: 2 adult tablets daily *31–40 kg*: 3 adult tablets daily *>40 kg*: 4 adult tablets (1 g atovaquone plus 400 mg proguanil) daily	No data, not recommended	No data, not recommended	Apparently safe in children >5 kg, but limited data	Hypersensitivity to atovaquone and/or proguanil; severe renal insufficiency (creatinine clearance <30 ml/min)	Take with food or milk drink to increase abosrption. Plasma concentrations of atovaquone are reduced when the drug is co-administered with rifampicin, rifabutin, metoclopramide or tetracycline. May interfere with live typhoid vaccine.
Choroquine	25 mg base/kg divided in daily dose (10, 10, 5 mg base/kg) for 3 days	Safe	Safe	Safe	Hypersensitivity to chloroquine; history of epilepsy; psoriasis	Use only for malaria caused by *P. vivax, P. ovale, P. malariae* or *P. knowlesi.* Concurrent use of chloroquine may reduce the antibody response to intradermally administered human diploid-cell rabies vaccine.

[a] See package insert for full information on contraindications and precautions.

Table 7.3 Use of antimalarial drugs for treatment of uncomplicated malaria in travellers (continued)

Generic name	Dosage regimen	Use in special groups			Main contraindications[a]	Comments[a]
		Pregnancy	Breast-feeding	Children		
Clindamycin	Under 60 kg: 5 mg base/kg 4 times daily for 5 days ≥60 kg: 300 mg base 4 times daily for 5 days	Apparently safe but limited data	Apparently safe but limited data	Apparently safe but limited data	Hypersensitivity to clindamycin or lincomycin; history of gastro-intestinal disease, particularly colitis; severe liver or kidney impairment.	Used in combination with quinine in areas of emerging quinine resistance.
Dihydro-artemisinin-piperaquine	One dose daily for 3 consecutive days. Target dose = 4 mg/kg per day dihydroartemisinin and 18 mg/kg per day piperaquine Adults >50 kg: 3 tablets daily for 3 days	No data, not recom-mended	No data, not recom-mended	Apparently safe in children >10 kg but limited data	Hypersensitivity to dihydroarte-misinin and/or piperaquine	Newer antimalarial medicine, submitted to the European Medicines Agency for regulatory approval in July 2009.
Doxycycline	Adults >50 kg: 800 mg salt over 7 days, taken as 2 tablets (100 mg salt each) 12 h apart on day 1, followed by 1 tablet daily for 6 days Children 8 years and older: 25–35 kg: 0.5 tablet per dose 36–50 kg: 0.75 tablet per dose >50 kg: 1 tablet per dose	Contra-indicated	Contra-indicated	Contra-indicated under 8 years of age	Hypersensitivity to tetracyclines; liver dysfunction.	Used in combination with quinine in areas of emerging quinine resistance.

[a] See package insert for full information on contraindications and precautions.

Table 7.3 Use of antimalarial drugs for treatment of uncomplicated malaria in travellers *(continued)*

Generic name	Dosage regimen	Use in special groups			Main contraindications[a]	Comments[a]
		Pregnancy	Breast-feeding	Children		
Mefloquine	25 mg base/kg as split dose (15 mg/kg plus 10 mg/kg 6–24 h apart)	Not recommended in first trimester because of lack of data	Safe	Not recommended under 5 kg because of lack of data	Hypersensitivity to mefloquine; psychiatric (including depression) or convulsive disorders; history of severe neuropsychiatric disease; concomitant halofantrine treatment; treatment with mefloquine in previous 4 weeks	Do not give mefloquine within 12 h of last dose of quinine treatment. Mefloquine and other related compounds (such as quinine, quinidine, chloroquine) may be given concomitantly only under close medical supervision because of possible additive cardiac toxicity and increased risk of convulsions; co-administration of mefloquine with anti-arrhythmic agents, beta-adrenergic blocking agents, calcium channel blockers, antihistamines including H1-blocking agents, and phenothiazines may contribute to prolongation of QTc interval. Ampicillin, tetracycline and metoclopramide may increase mefloquine blood levels.
Primaquine	0.25 mg base/kg, taken with food once daily for 14 days. In Oceania and south-east Asia the dose should be 0.5 mg base/kg	Contraindicated	Contraindicated unless infant has been determined NOT to be G6PD deficient	Lower age limit not established. Generally contraindicated in young infants	G6PD deficiency; active rheumatoid arthritis; lupus erythematosus; conditions that predispose to granulocytopenia; concomitant use of drugs that may induce haematological disorders	Used as anti-relapse treatment for *P. vivax* and *P. ovale* infections.

[a] See package insert for full information on contraindications and precautions.

Table 7.3 Use of antimalarial drugs for treatment of uncomplicated malaria in travellers *(continued)*

| Generic name | Dosage regimen | Use in special groups | | | Main contraindications[a] | Comments[a] |
		Pregnancy	Breast-feeding	Children		
Quinine	8 mg base/kg 3 times daily for 7 days	Safe	Safe	Safe	Hypersensitivity to quinine or quinidine; tinnitus; optic neuritis; haemolysis; myasthenia gravis. Use with caution in persons with G6PD deficiency and in patients with atrial fibrillation, cardiac conduction defects or heart block. Quinine may enhance effect of cardiosuppressant drugs. Use with caution in persons using beta-blockers, digoxin, calcium channel blockers, etc.	In areas of emerging resistance to quinine, give in combination with doxycycline, tetracycline or clindamycin. Quinine may induce hypoglycaemia, particularly in (malnourished) children, pregnant women and patients with severe disease.

[a] See package insert for full information on contraindications and precautions.

7.5 Countries and territories with malarious areas

The following list shows all countries/territories where malaria occurs. In some of these countries/territories, malaria is present only in certain areas or up to a particular altitude. In many countries, malaria has a seasonal pattern. These details as well as information on the predominant malaria species, status of resistance to antimalarial drugs and recommended type of prevention are provided in the Country list.

(* = *P. vivax* risk only)

Afghanistan
Algeria*
Angola
Argentina*
Armenia*
Azerbaijan*
Bahamas
Bangladesh
Belize
Benin
Bhutan
Bolivia, Plurinational
    State of
Botswana
Brazil
Burkina Faso
Burundi
Cambodia
Cameroon
Cape Verde
Central African
    Republic
Chad
China
Colombia
Comoros
Congo
Congo, Democratic
    Republic of the
    (former Zaire)
Costa Rica
Côte d'Ivoire
Djibouti
Dominican Republic
Ecuador
Egypt
El Salvador
Equatorial Guinea
Eritrea
Ethiopia

French Guiana
Gabon
Gambia
Georgia*
Ghana
Guatemala
Guinea
Guinea-Bissau
Guyana
Haiti
Honduras
India
Indonesia
Iran, Islamic Republic of
Iraq*
Jamaica
Kenya
Korea, Democratic
    People's Republic of*
Korea, Republic of*
Kyrgyzstan*
Lao People's Democratic
    Republic
Liberia
Madagascar
Malawi
Malaysia
Mali
Mauritania
Mayotte
Mexico
Mozambique
Myanmar
Namibia
Nepal
Nicaragua
Niger
Nigeria
Oman
Pakistan

Panama
Papua New Guinea
Paraguay*
Peru
Philippines
Russian Federation*
Rwanda
Sao Tome and Principe
Saudi Arabia
Senegal
Sierra Leone
Solomon Islands
Somalia
South Africa
Sri Lanka
Sudan
Suriname
Swaziland
Syrian Arab
    Republic*
Tajikistan
Thailand
Timor-Leste
Togo
Turkey*
Uganda
United Republic
    of Tanzania
Uzbekistan*
Vanuatu
Venezuela, Bolivarian
    Republic of
Viet Nam
Yemen
Zambia
Zimbabwe

Further reading

Guidelines for the treatment of malaria, 2nd ed. Geneva, World Health Organization, 2010.

Malaria vector control and personal protection: report of a WHO Study Group. Geneva, World Health Organization, 2006 (WHO Technical Report Series, No. 936).

Management of severe malaria: a practical handbook, 2nd ed. Geneva, World Health Organization, 2000.

These documents are available on the WHO Global Malaria Programme web site: http://www.who.int/malaria.

CHAPTER 8

Exposure to blood or other body fluids

8.1 Blood transfusion

Blood transfusion is a life-saving intervention. When used correctly, it saves lives and improves health. However, blood transfusion carries a potential risk of acute or delayed reactions and transfusion-transmissible infections and should be prescribed only to treat conditions associated with significant morbidity that cannot be prevented or managed effectively by other means.

For travellers, the need for a blood transfusion almost always arises as a result of a medical emergency involving sudden massive blood loss, such as:

- accidental injury, such as road traffic accident
- gynaecological or obstetric emergency
- severe gastrointestinal haemorrhage
- emergency surgery.

The safety of blood and blood products depends on the following key factors:

- A supply of safe blood and blood products through the careful selection of voluntary unpaid blood donors from low-risk populations who donate regularly, testing all donated blood for transfusion-transmissible infections, and correct storage and transportation at all stages from collection to transfusion within an adequate quality system.

- Appropriate prescription (only when there is no other remedy), proper cross-matching between the blood unit and the recipient, and safe administration of the blood or blood product at the bedside, with correct patient identification.

In many developing countries, safe blood and blood products may not be available in all health care facilities. In addition, evidence from every region of the world indicates considerable variations in patterns of clinical blood use between different hospitals, different clinical specialities and even between different clinicians within the same speciality. This suggests that blood and blood products are often transfused unnecessarily.

While blood transfusions given correctly save millions of lives every year, unsafe blood transfusions – as a result of the incompatibility of the blood, the volume transfused or the transmission of infections such as hepatitis B, hepatitis C, HIV, malaria, syphilis or Chagas disease – can lead to serious reactions in the recipients.

The initial management of major haemorrhage is the prevention of further blood loss and restoration of the blood volume as rapidly as possible in order to maintain tissue perfusion and oxygenation. This requires infusing the patient with large volumes of replacement fluids until the haemorrhage can be controlled. Some patients respond quickly and remain stable following the infusion of crystalloids or colloids and may not require blood transfusion.

In malaria-endemic areas, there is a high risk of acquiring malaria from transfusion. It may be necessary to administer the routine treatment for malaria to the transfused patients (Chapter 7).

Precautions

- Travellers should carry a medical card or other document showing their blood group and information about any current medical problems or treatment.

- Unnecessary travel should be avoided by those with pre-existing conditions that may give rise to a need for blood transfusion.

- Those on treatment of anaemia, should carry and take required medications to avoid worsening of anaemia.

- Travellers should take all possible precautions to avoid involvement in traffic accidents or other accidental injuries (Chapter 4).

- Travellers should obtain a contact address at the travel destination, in advance, for advice and assistance in case of medical emergency.

- Travellers should discuss with attending physician on the use of alternatives to transfusion, if the need arises.

- Travellers with chronic medical conditions such as thalassaemia or haemophilia, which necessitate regular transfusion of blood or plasma-derived products, should obtain medical advice on the management of their condition before travelling. They should also identify appropriate medical facilities at their travel destination and carry a supply of the relevant safe products with them, if appropriate.

8.2 Accidental exposure to blood or other body fluids

Exposure to bloodborne pathogens may occur in case of:

- contact between blood or body fluids and a non-intact skin or with mucous membranes;
- percutaneous injury with needles or sharp instruments contaminated with blood or body fluids.

These exposures may occur:

- when using contaminated syringes and needles for injecting drugs;
- as a result of accidents or acts of violence, including sexual assaults;
- in case of sexual exposure if no condom was used, or if the condom was broken;
- as occupational exposure, within and outside health care settings, to health care and other workers (such as rescuers, police officers) in the course of the work or to patients;
- during natural or man-made disasters.

Accidental exposure may lead to infection by bloodborne pathogens, particularly hepatitis B, hepatitis C and HIV. The average risk of seroconversion after a single percutaneous exposure to infected blood is approximately 2% for hepatitis C and 6–60% for hepatitis B. For HIV, the average risk of seroconversion after a single percutaneous exposure to HIV-infected blood is 0.1–0.3%.

Pre-exposure vaccination. Hepatitis B vaccination can be given before exposure to protect travellers from hepatitis B infection (Chapter 6). There are no vaccines for hepatitis C or HIV.

Post-exposure prophylaxis. Post-exposure prophylaxis (PEP) is an emergency medical response given as soon as possible after potential exposure to reduce the risk of transmission of bloodborne pathogens. It is available for HIV and hepatitis B.

Accidental exposure to potentially infected blood or other body fluids is a medical emergency. The following measures should be taken without delay:

1. Immediate first-aid care.

2. Refer to a service provider and report the accident.

3. PEP, if applicable.

8.2.1 First-aid care management of exposure to bloodborne pathogens

After percutaneous exposure

- Allow the wound to bleed freely.
- Do not squeeze or rub the injury site.
- Wash site immediately using soap and water that will not irritate the skin.
- If running water is not available, clean site with hand-cleaning solution or gel.
- Do not use any strong solutions, such as bleach, iodine or alcohol-based products, as these may irritate the wound and make the injury worse.

After a splash of blood or body fluids onto unbroken skin

- Wash the area immediately with running water.
- If running water is not available, clean the area with any hand-cleaning solution.
- Do not use alcohol-based antiseptics.
- Do not rub the skin.

After exposure of the eye

- Irrigate the exposed eye immediately with a sterile eye solution, water or normal saline.
- Sit in a chair, tilt the head back and ask someone to gently pour water or normal saline over the eye, gently pulling the eyelids up and down to make sure the eye is cleaned thoroughly.
- If wearing contact lenses, leave them in place while irrigating, as they form a barrier over the eye and will help protect it. Once the eye has been cleaned, remove the contact lenses and clean them in the normal manner. This will make them safe to wear again.
- **Do not** use soap or disinfectant on the eye.

After exposure of the mouth

- Spit the fluid out immediately.
- Rinse the mouth thoroughly, using water or normal saline, and spit out again. Repeat this process several times.

- **Do not** use soap or disinfectant in the mouth.

In all cases, a health care worker should be contacted immediately.

Post-exposure prophylaxis (PEP)

HIV

For HIV, PEP refers to a set of comprehensive services to prevent HIV infection in the exposed individual. These services include risk assessment and counselling, HIV testing based on informed consent and – according to the risk assessment – the provision of short-term antiretroviral (ARV) drugs, with follow-up and support. Counselling and risk assessment are critical before providing PEP for HIV. HIV testing is strongly recommended for both the exposed individual and the source individual (if known). Testing should never be mandatory or conditional for PEP; any case should be supported with appropriate counselling and the provision of PEP should be based on informed consent. Other tests (hepatitis B, hepatitis C and screening for sexually transmitted diseases in the case of sexual exposure) may be indicated.

PEP should be started as soon as possible after the incident and ideally within less than 2 h. The decision to provide ARV drugs depends on a number of factors, including the HIV status of the exposed and source person (if known), the nature of the body fluid involved, the severity of exposure and the period between exposure and the beginning of treatment. PEP should not be given to people who test or are known to be HIV-positive.

The recommended PEP regimen is, in most cases, a combination of two ARV drugs that should be taken continuously for 28 days. In some instances, when drug resistance may be suspected in the source person, a third drug may be added. Expert consultation is especially important when exposure to drug-resistant HIV may have occurred. More information is available at: http://www.who.int/hiv/topics/prophylaxis/en/.

If an initial HIV test has been done, subsequent tests should be repeated at 8 weeks after exposure and at 6 months if ARVs have been taken. People who test positive at any stage should be offered psychological support and appropriate treatment when needed.

Even when taking ARVs for PEP after exposure to HIV infection, the exposed individual should not have unprotected sexual intercourse or donate blood until the 6-month post-exposure tests confirm that he or she is not seropositive. Women should avoid becoming pregnant during this period. Breastfeeding should be discussed with a service provider and avoided if safe alternatives exist.

Hepatitis B

Recommended post-exposure management algorithms for testing and administration of hepatitis B vaccine and/or hepatitis B immune globulin should be followed.

Hepatitis C

People exposed to hepatitis C virus may be screened for hepatitis C virus RNA at baseline, 4–6 weeks and 4–6 months after exposure.

Hepatitis E

People exposed to hepatitis E virus may be screened for anti-HEV IgM antibodies or for hepatitis E virus RNA.

Further reading

Post-exposure prophylaxis for HIV: http://www.who.int/hiv/topics/prophylaxis/en/

Updated U.S. Public Health Service guidelines for the management of occupational exposures to HBV, HCV, and HIV and recommendations for postexposure prophylaxis. *Morbidity and Mortality Weekly Report*, 2001, 50(RR-11) (available at: http://www.cdc.gov/mmwr/PDF/rr/rr5011.pdf).

Special groups of travellers

9.1 Travel to visit friends and relatives

According to the United Nations, international migration rose from 120 million in 1990 to more than 200 million in 2006. In many countries immigrants now constitute more than 20% of the population. Immigrants increasingly travel to their place of origin to visit friends and relatives (VFR), and VFR travel is now a major component of the international journeys that take place annually. The term "VFRs" generally refers to immigrants from a developing country to an industrialized country who subsequently return to their home countries for the purpose of visiting friends and relatives.

Compared with tourists to the same destinations, VFRs are at increased risk of travel-related diseases. These include – but are not limited to – malaria, hepatitis A and B, typhoid fever, rabies, tuberculosis, and the diseases normally preventable by routine childhood immunization. For example, the global surveillance data of GeoSentinel (an international network of travel medicine providers) on returned travel patients show that eight times more VFR travellers than tourists present with malaria as their diagnosed illness. It is estimated that VFRs account for more than half the total imported malaria cases in Europe and North America.

The greater risk for VFRs is related to a number of factors, including higher risk of exposure and insufficient protective measures. These individuals are less likely to seek pre-travel advice or to be adequately vaccinated, but more likely to stay in remote rural areas, have close contact with local populations, consume high-risk food and beverages, undertake last-minute travel (linked to deaths or other family emergencies) and make trips of greater duration. Because of familiarity with their place of origin, VFRs may perceive less risk, which may result in lower rates of pre-departure vaccinations or malaria prophylaxis. The cost of pre-travel consultation, often not covered by health insurance programmes, may be onerous for VFRs, in particular those with large families, and access to travel medicine services may be hampered by cultural and linguistic limitations.

Improving the access of VFRs to pre-travel health counselling is of increasing public health importance. Primary health-care providers need to become more aware of the increased risks faced by VFRs. Strategies are needed to increase the awareness among VFRs of travel-related health risks and to facilitate uptake of pre-travel health advice, vaccinations and, where indicated, malaria prophylaxis.

9.2 Mass gatherings

The term "mass gathering" is used for any assembly of more than 1000 people at a specific location, for a specific purpose, for a period of time. These include sporting events (e.g. the Olympic Games), cultural events (e.g. world exhibitions, music festivals) social events (e.g. national day gatherings) and religious gatherings and pilgrimages. With increasing air travel and globalization, mass gatherings – while varying in size and nature and purpose – present diverse public health challenges. Health hazards may be increased as a result of the concentration of people in enclosed and non-enclosed events.

Factors associated with increased risk of health hazards are the following:

- influx of large numbers of visitors within a short period of time;
- visitors often come from areas that differ greatly in both geography and culture;
- conditions of overcrowding;

In planning for a mass gathering, organizers should complete a risk assessment for public health threats. Measures to address and manage the public health risks should be identified, including:

- public health surveillance;
- outbreak detection and diagnostic resources;
- communications systems;
- response (including quarantine or isolation facilities) and emergency resources; and
- medical resources (including pharmaceuticals and equipment).

Public health planning usually involves a range of organizations within the context of international, federal and local laws and regulations. Security and law enforcement authorities should also be involved in the planning for public health security, which includes planning for infectious disease control measures, natural disaster and medical intervention, awareness and vigilance.

WHO has convened several technical workshops on mass gatherings.[1] The resulting guidelines address the assessment of relevant public health risks; evaluation of the capacity of existing systems and services, in anticipation of the surge of public health needs of mass gatherings; and development of control systems for biosurveillance, emergency response, crowd control, disease outbreak detection and response, laboratory services, mass communications, preparations for potential quarantine control, and management of mass casualties.

Hajj, a religious pilgrimage and mass gathering

Data for quantifying the risk of medical problems related to religious pilgrimages are limited; the best documented, in terms of health risk, is the Hajj, the annual Muslim pilgrimage to Mecca and Medina in Saudi Arabia.

In scale and international diversity, the Hajj is a unique religious pilgrimage. It is undertaken by Muslims as a once-in-a -lifetime act of religious devotion during the days of the Hajj; the Umrah is a similar pilgrimage undertaken at other times of the year.

During the Hajj, more than 2 million Muslims from all over the world congregate to perform their religious rituals. The resulting overcrowding has led to stampedes, traffic accidents and fire injuries. Cardiovascular disease is the most common cause of death. Heatstroke and severe dehydration are also frequent when the Hajj season falls during the summer months. The potential for spread of infectious diseases associated with this pilgrimage has long been recognized. Throughout its 14-century history, the Hajj has been associated with major health issues: historical records document outbreaks of plague and cholera, involving large numbers of pilgrims, when quarantine was the prime means of control.

Each year, the date of Hajj is 10 or 11 days earlier than in the previous year, since it is dictated by the Islamic lunar calendar. Thus different seasonal conditions prevail during the Hajj and may be favourable to different diseases, such as influenza or dengue fever. Overcrowding also contributes to the potential dissemination of airborne infectious diseases or infections associated with person-to-person transmission. Extensive outbreaks of meningococcal disease among pilgrims have prompted the Saudi Arabian health authorities to introduce mandatory vaccination. All pilgrims must now be given the quadrivalent meningococcal vaccine (protecting against serogroups A, C, Y and W-135). The most frequently reported complaints

---

[1] *Communicable disease alert and response for mass gatherings: key considerations.* Geneva, World Health Organization, 2008 (available at: http://www.who.int/csr/Mass_gatherings2. pdf).

among pilgrims are upper respiratory symptoms. Seasonal influenza vaccination has been reported to reduce influenza-like illness among pilgrims and should be a highly recommended vaccination for all those making the Hajj, particularly those with pre-existing conditions (e.g. the elderly, people with chronic chest or heart diseases as well as hepatic or renal failure). Pneumococcal vaccination should also be recommended for those aged over 65 years and those who would benefit from it because of underlying medical conditions (Chapter 6).

Hajj-related outbreaks of cholera occurred in the past, but not since 1989 following improvements to the water supply and sewage systems. Hepatitis A vaccination is recommended for non-immune pilgrims, and routine vaccinations (such as poliomyelitis, tetanus, diphtheria and hepatitis B (Chapter 6)) should be up to date. Yellow fever vaccine is a requirement for pilgrims coming from areas or countries with risk of transmission of yellow fever (Annex 1).

The Ministry of Health of Saudi Arabia requires all travellers arriving from countries or areas reporting indigenous wild polio viruses (in 2010: Afghanistan, India, Nigeria and Pakistan) be vaccinated with oral polio vaccine (OPV) at least 6 weeks before application for entry visa (Chapter 6). In addition, travellers under 15 years of age arriving from countries or areas reporting imported wild polio virus (updates available at http://www.polioeradication.org/Dataandmonitoring/Poliothisweek. aspx) are also subject to the same entry visa requirement (Chapter 6).

All of the above travellers arriving in Saudi Arabia will also receive OPV at border points.

Updates on requirements and recommendations for the annual Hajj pilgrimage can be found in the *Weekly Epidemiological Record* (available on line at http://www.who.int/wer/en).

9.3 Travellers with HIV/AIDS

As a result of improved health and prognosis, HIV-infected individuals are increasingly likely to engage in travel-related activities that may expose them to other diseases.

9.3.1 Special issues for HIV-infected travellers

- Increased susceptibility/morbidity to many tropical infections
- Vaccines:
    - reduced immune response to some vaccines

— risk of severe adverse reactions to live vaccines
- Drug interactions
- Country travel restrictions based on HIV status
- Access to medical resources during travel

9.3.2 The natural course of HIV infection

The natural course of infection with HIV is characterized by chronic replication of HIV as measured by plasma HIV-RNA and leads to progressive immunodeficiency characterized by a decline of CD4 lymphocyte counts in peripheral blood. Pre-travel advice therefore also depends on CD4 lymphocyte counts (Table 9.1).

9.3.3 Antiretroviral therapy

Antiretroviral therapy (ART) inhibits HIV replication (plasma HIV-RNA becomes undetectable) and leads to a partial restoration of immunocompetence (rise in CD4 counts). ART usually includes three antiretroviral drugs. Rigorous adherence to ART is essential to avoid development of resistance and treatment should not be interrupted.

Pre-travel assessments include risks associated with travel itinerary, current ART, current CD4 counts and plasma HIV-RNA, medical history and physical examination.

Travellers should ideally be on a stable ART regimen for 3 months before undertaking long journeys and plasma HIV-RNA (if available) should be undetectable. Newly diagnosed individuals with CD4 cell counts $<200/mm^3$ may wish to delay travel until counts have improved with ART, particularly if they are travelling to countries where hygiene, sanitation and medical care are inadequate. This delay will minimize the risk of travel-associated infections, of immune reconstitution inflammatory syndrome during travel and allows time to observe the tolerability and efficacy of antiretroviral drugs.

Disruption of daily routines related to travel have been associated with reduced adherence to ARV treatment or prophylaxis treatment for one or more opportunistic infections (e.g. pneumocystis, mycobacteria, toxoplasma) and this should be discussed with the individual.

Adaptation of the dosing schedule is needed if the journey includes change of time zones. Intervals between doses should preferably be shortened, not lengthened. Timing can generally be adjusted plus or minus one hour per day until the desired convenient dosing time is reached. For short trips (1–2 weeks), it may be simpler to maintain the same dosing time as at home. There are no special storage requirements for other antiretrovirals which can be stored at ambient room temperature.

Travellers should understand that if it is necessary to stop ART (e.g. in the case of drug stock-outs caused by emergency situations such as natural disasters or civil disturbance) and the patient is taking a NRTI/NNRTI combination,[2] the NNRTI (efavirenz or nevirapine) should be stopped first and the two NRTIs continued for 7 days and then stopped. This "staggered stopping" reduces the significant risk (up to 60%) of NNRTI resistance observed if all three drugs are stopped at the same time.

Table 9.1 **Pre-travel counselling according to CD4 count**

CD4 count	Important counselling points
>350/mm³	Food and water hygiene If on ART: interactions, adherence Izoniazid prophylaxis for tuberculosis if indicated.
200-350/mm³	Food and water hygiene ART indicated If of ART: interactions, adherence If not on successful ART: consider pneumocystis prophylaxis for longer travels Izoniazid prophylaxis for tuberculosis if indicated Vaccine efficacy reduced Yellow fever vaccination: avoid unless high-risk of exposure
<200/mm³	Food and water hygiene Risk for opportunistic infections, ART and co-trimoxazole for theco trimoxazole primary prophylaxis of pneumocystis and bacterial diarrheadiarrhoea and toxoplasmosis indicated Izoniazid prophylaxis for tuberculosis if indicated Vaccine efficacy reduced Avoid yellow fever vaccine Consider delaying longer journeys until after several months of successful ART and CD4 count above 200/ mm³ If on ART: interactions, adherence
<50/mm³	Food and water hygiene High risk for all opportunistic infections, ART and Coco-trimoxazole for the primary prophylaxis of pneumocystis and bacterial indicated Vaccine efficacy severely reduced Avoid yellow fever vaccine Delay longer journeys until after several months of successful ART and CD4 count >200/ mm³ If on ART: interactions, adherence

---

[2] Nucleoside reverse transcriptase inhibitor/non-nucleoside reverse transcriptase inhibitor.

Many antiretroviral drugs interact with other drugs and this must be taken into account when advising travellers on malaria prophylaxis and other drugs.

Travellers need to be reminded that Ritonavir capsules should be kept refrigerated but can be kept at room temperature (<25 °C) for a maximum of 28 days and that there are no special storage requirements for other antiretrovirals, which can be stored at ambient room temperature.

Finally, travellers should carry a document certifying their need for the prescribed life-saving drugs but that makes no mention of HIV infection. They are advised to carry several days doses of ART in their hand-luggage.

9.3.4 Travel restrictions

Some countries have introduced various restrictions on entry, stay, residency or activities for international travellers with HIV infection. HIV-infected travellers are advised to obtain authoritative information on these issues from relevant embassies, consulates, missions or other appropriate sources.

9.3.5 Medical resources abroad

HIV-infected travellers should have medical insurance that includes coverage abroad, emergency assistance and repatriation. They should carry a medical report and should be informed about medical resources abroad. A useful list of more than 3300 organizations in 175 countries involved in counselling and care of HIV-infected individuals is provided by a non-profit community-based HIV information provider, the National AIDS Manual (NAM), and can be found at www.aidsmap.com.

9.3.6 Increased susceptibility to selected pathogens and morbidity risk

With falling CD4 counts, HIV-infected individuals are more susceptible to many pathogens and are at higher risk for more severe disease. Infections that are often self-limiting in immunocompetent hosts may become chronic and severe in HIV-infected individuals. Preventing exposure is therefore important, since vaccines are available for only a limited number of the pathogens and their immunogenicity may be reduced in the most vulnerable patients.

Travellers' diarrhoea
HIV-infected patients are more susceptible to most foodborne and waterborne pathogens. Morbidity and mortality may be higher, e.g. non-typhoidal salmonellae often cause invasive infections in patients with severe immunodeficiency. Proto-

zoa such as *Cryptosporidium, Isospora, Cyclospora* and species of microsporidia), which cause self-limiting diarrhoea in immmunocompetent travellers, may cause chronic and devastating opportunistic disease in immunodeficient patients. Food hygiene is therefore critical (Chapter 3).

In febrile or dysenteric diarrhoea emergencies when travelling to remote areas, HIV-infected patients with moderate to severe immunodeficiency should carry empirical stand-by antibiotic treatment with full information on its use. The antibiotics prescribed must take account of the resistance patterns of *Salmonella, Shigella, Escherichia coli* and *Campylobacter* in the region of travel. Fluoroquinolones and co-trimoxazole are active against several enteric pathogens and do not interact significantly with ART. Azithromycin is also a good choice, particularly for those travelling to Asia. However, other macrolide antibiotics may have significant interactions with ART that should be taken into account if used. Patients should seek specialized care if symptoms do not improve within 24–48 h.

Tuberculosis
HIV infection is associated with a higher risk of developing active tuberculosis after exposure to, or reactivation of latent infection with, *Mycobacterium tuberculosis*. HIV-infected travellers should be assessed for latent tuberculosis infection and close (household) exposure to tuberculosis and treated with isoniazid preventive therapy (IPT), provided that active tuberculosis is excluded. BCG vaccine should *not* be given, regardless of whether these HIV-positive individuals are symptomatic or asymptomatic.

Other pathogens
Greater susceptibility and/or morbidity is also important in the case of Leishmania (a protozoan infection transmitted by the sandfly), malaria (transmitted by mosquito bites), Trypanosoma, and fungi, especially histoplasmosis, coccidioidomycosis (Americas) and *Penicillium marneffei* (South-East Asia). Preventive measures include use of (impregnated) mosquito nets, coils and repellents, prevention of arthropod bites and avoidance of sites with high exposure such as areas of stagnant water, bat and bird caves.

9.3.7 Vaccines
The basic principles of vaccination that apply to all travellers in terms of timing, dosing, assessment of antibody responses (Chapter 6) apply also to HIV-infected individuals. Differences for individual vaccines are summarized in Table 9.2.

Table 9.2 **Pre-exposure vaccines for HIV-infected travellers**

Vaccine	Indication	Notes
Live vaccines		
Influenza (intranasal)	Contraindicated	Use inactivated parenteral vaccine Avoid vaccination in household contacts
Japanese encephalitis (SA-14-14-2)	Contraindicated	
Measles/mumps/rubella (MMR)	Indicated for measles in IgG-seronegative travellers with CD4 count >200 cells/ mm^3 Contraindicated in travellers with CD4 ≤200 cells/ mm^3	Avoid pregnancy for 1 month after vaccination Breastfeeding not contraindicated Administer 2 doses at least 1 month apart to increase likelihood of protection against measles No data suggest increased adverse events following measles vaccination of HIV-infected children, but efficacy may be impaired for mumps and rubella. Household contacts can be vaccinated
Poliomyelitis, oral (OPV)	Indicated	Polio vaccination indicated for all travellers to countries or areas reporting wild polio viruses (see http://www.who.polioeradication.org/ casecount.asp). Travellers who have previously received three or more doses of OPV or IPV should be offered another dose of vaccine before departure. Non-immunized individuals require a complete course of vaccination. OPV is not contraindicated in HIV-infected children. For the purposes of travellers' vaccination, OPV or IPV can be used in asymptomatic HIV-infected individuals.
Tuberculosis (BCG)	Contraindicated	

Vaccine	Indication	Notes
Typhoid (Ty21a)	Indicated for HIV-infected individuals with CD4 counts >200 cells/ mm^3	Consider inactivated typhoid ViCPS vaccine
Varicella	Varicella indicated for varicella-seronegative patients with CD3 count >200 cells/mm^3	Pregnancy should be avoided for 1 month following vaccination
Yellow fever (YF)	Indicated if significant risk of YF for travellers with CD4 count >200 cells/ mm^3, whether or not on ART Contraindicated in HIV-infected travellers with CD4 ≤200 cells/ mm^3 on CCR5 inhibitors[a]	Decisions regarding YF vaccination should always be taken in light of likely risk of acquisition of infection An exemption certificate should be provided to individuals with a contraindication to the YF vaccine travelling to countries or areas at risk of YF Advice on avoidance of mosquito bites

Inactivated vaccines/toxoids

Vaccine	Indication	Notes
Cholera (WC/rBS)	Indicated for travellers to high-risk areas during epidemics or after natural disasters	Limited efficacy and safety data Also induces protection against enterotoxigenic *Escherichia coli* (ETEC) Responses in travellers with CD4 <100 cells/mm^3 are poor Stress good food and water hygiene
Diphtheria/tetanus/pertussis	Indicated	
Hepatitis A	Indicated for non-immune travellers to countries or areas at risk, particularly those in high-risk groups[b]	If resources allow, check for serological evidence of natural infection before vaccination Serological responses reduced in immunosuppressed patients, but good efficacy even at low CD4 count Two or three doses required Consider human normal immunoglobulin(HNIG) for severely immunosuppressed travellers

Vaccine	Indication	Notes
		May be given as single vaccine or as combination with hepatitis B
Hepatitis B	Recommended for all non-immune, susceptible travellers	3-dose schedule (0,1,2–12 months) ± booster doses as dictated by serological response Those who fail to respond to 1st vaccination course (as indicated by anti-HBs<10 mIU/ml) should receive a 2nd course Stress advice on risk reduction, especially in high-risk groups such as men who have sex with men
Seasonal Influenza vaccine	Indicated	Inactivated parenteral vaccine is recommended at the start of the influenza season
Japanese encephalitis (JE)	Indicated for long-term travellers to south-east Asia and western Pacific and for those with extensive exposure to rural areas of these regions even if travelling short-term (see Chapter 6)	Formalin-inactivated JE virus vaccine derived from mouse brains has been linked with severe neurological adverse events requiring careful evaluation of the traveller's risk and need for vaccination A new inactivated JE virus vaccine (Chapter 6) has recently been licensed in several countries, but no information is available yet for HIV-infected individuals
Neisseria meningitidis	Mandatory vaccine for Hajj pilgrims; indicated for travellers to the "meningitis belt"	Quadrivalent (ACWY) vaccine recommended No evidence of increased risk of adverse events in HIV-infected individuals
Poliomyelitis, injectable (IPV)	Indicated	Polio vaccination indicated for all travellers to countries or areas reporting wild polio viruses (see http://www.polioeradication.org/casecount.asp). Travellers who have previously received three or more doses of OPV or IPV should be offered another dose of vaccine

Vaccine	Indication	Notes
		before departure. Non-immunized individuals require a complete course of vaccination.
Rabies	Indicated for travellers who could be exposed to rabid animals (Chapter 6 and Map)	Intramuscular immunization recommended rather than intradermal Assess response to immunization in travellers with CD4 cells ≤200/mm³, if resources allow, ± further boosting if antibody response >0.5IU/ml not achieved Counsel all travellers to countries or areas at risk on wound treatment and post-exposure prophylaxis
Tick-borne encephalitis	Indicated for HIV-infected travellers intending to walk, camp or work in heavily forested regions in areas at risk	Limited efficacy data available; travellers with CD4 count >400 cells/mm³ generally have better serological response Highest risk in late spring/early summer Stress importance of avoiding tick bites and consumption of unpasteurized milk
Typhoid (ViCPS)	Indicated for HIV-infected travellers at risk of exposure, particularly in high risk areas	Booster every 3 years Serological response reduced in travellers with CD4 count ≤200 cells/mm³ Stress food and water hygiene

[a] A severe viscerotropic disease after YF vaccination has been described in an HIV-negative individual with genetically determined disruption of the CCR5 RANTES axis.

[b] Men who have sex with men, intravenous drug users, haemophiliacs receiving plasma-derived concentrates and patients with hepatitis B and/or C co-infection.

Immunogenicity

Low CD4 counts and replicating HIV infection are associated with a reduced immunogenicity of most vaccines. Antibody titres after vaccination are lower shortly after vaccination and decline more rapidly, particularly in patients with CD4 counts below 200/mm3. If feasible, vaccination against travel-associated diseases should be postponed until successful ART has led to a sustained increase in CD4 counts (ideally above 350/mm3). Some vaccine courses will require extra or booster doses, depending on the individual vaccine. If exposure cannot be postponed, inactivated vaccines should be given if indicated, even in patients with low CD4 counts, and revaccination should be performed after immune restoration.

Vaccine safety

Inactivated vaccines are safe in HIV-infected individuals. In general, HIV-infected travellers should avoid live vaccines, although yellow fever and measles/mumps/rubella (MMR) may be given to patients with CD4 cell counts >200/mm^3.

9.3.8 Malaria in HIV-infected travellers

Worsening HIV-related immunosuppression may lead to increasing parasite burdens and more severe manifestations of malaria. Like all travellers, immunocompromised individuals travelling to countries or areas at risk of malaria transmission should be protected against malaria and be aware of the risks, be prescribed appropriate drugs for malaria chemoprophylaxis and given clear advice about avoidance of mosquito bites; they should immediately seek diagnosis and treatment if a fever develops (Chapters 3 and 7).

Chemoprophylaxis should preferably be started well before travelling as adverse events may necessitate a change in regimen. Compliance with malaria prophylaxis, early treatment-seeking (within 24 h of onset of any febrile illness), prompt definitive diagnosis (using malaria smears or rapid diagnostic tests) and effective treatment are particularly important in HIV-infected patients. Travellers with HIV infection who develop malaria should receive prompt, effective antimalarial treatment in line with the recommendations for international travellers (Chapter 7).

HIV-infected patients may be receiving other medications, such as co-trimoxazole (trimethoprim–sulfamethoxazole) as prophylaxis for opportunistic infections, and/or ART. There is limited information on drug interactions between ART and artemisinin-based combination therapy (ACT) for malaria. In one study, treatment of uncomplicated malaria with the ACT artesunate–amodiaquine was highly effective in both HIV-infected and uninfected children. Importantly, however, there was a significant 7–8-fold increase in the risk of neutropenia 14 days after initiation of treatment among HIV-infected children compared with uninfected children. About one-fifth of the episodes in the HIV-infected group were severe or life-threatening. Among the HIV-infected children, the risk of neutropenia was significantly higher among those on ART regimens containing zidovudine. Hepatotoxicity has been documented for efavirenz given together with artesunate–amodiaquine. Given this limited but worrying information, treatment of malaria in HIV-infected patients receiving zidovudine or efavirenz should, if possible, avoid ACT regimens containing amodiaquine. Information on possible interactions with other ACTs is also limited. Although HIV infection and co-trimoxazole may also depress neutrophil counts, there is insufficient information on the interaction of amodiaquine-containing ACT regimens with co-trimoxazole and HIV infection to allow recommendations to be made.

- Patients with HIV infection who develop malaria should receive prompt, effective antimalarial treatment regimens in line with the recommendations for international travellers (see Chapter 7).

- Treatment abroad with sulfadoxine–pyrimethamine-containing ACT regimens should be avoided in HIV-infected patients on co-trimoxazole (trimethoprim–sulfamethoxazole) prophylaxis.

- Treatment abroad with amodiaquine-containing ACT regimens should be avoided if possible in HIV-infected patients on zidovudine or efavirenz.

Further reading

Ahmed QA, Arabi YM, Memish ZA. Health risks at the Hajj. *Lancet*, 2006, 367:1008–1015.

Behrens RH, Barnett ED. Visiting friends and relatives. In: Keystone JS et al. eds. *Travel medicine*, 2nd ed. Edinburgh, Mosby, 2008, 291–298.

Geretti AM et al. British HIV Association guidelines for immunization of HIV-infected adults 2008. *HIV Medicine*, 2008, 9:795–848.

Guidelines for the treatment of malaria, 2nd edition. Geneva, World Health Organization, 2010.

Information on GeoSentinel: http://www.istm.org/geosentinel/main.html

International migration and development. Report of the Secretary General. New York, United Nations, 2006 (A60/871).

Leder K et al. Illness in travelers visiting friends and relatives: a review of the GeoSentinel Surveillance Network. *Clinical Infectious Diseases*, 2006, 43(9):1185–1193.

Tourism highlights: 2006 edition. Madrid, World Tourism Organization, 2006 (available at http://www.unwto.org/facts/menu.html).

Trends in total migrant stock: the 2005 revision. New York, Population Division, Department of Economic and Social Affairs, United Nations (available at: http://www.un.org/esa/population/publications/migration/UN_Migrant_Stock_Documentation_2005.pdf).

CHAPTER 10

Psychological health

10.1 General considerations

International travel is often a stressful experience. Travellers face separation from family and familiar social support systems, and must deal with the impact of foreign cultures and languages, as well as bewildering, unfamiliar threats to health and safety. Coping with high levels of stress may result in physical, social and psychological problems. Those who encounter a greater range of stress factors may be at greater risk for psychological problems. Under the stress of travel, pre-existing mental disorders can be exacerbated. Furthermore, for those people with a predisposition towards mental disorder, such a disorder may emerge for the first time during travel.

Physicians caring for people in their home countries or overseas should be aware of the differences (both within and between countries) in the availability of mental health resources (for example, emergency facilities, staff, beds and investigative facilities) as well as in the type and quality of medication. Culturally compatible clinicians and support staff may be rare or non-existent, and they may not understand the native language of the traveller, so access to interpreters may be necessary. The legal environment within which a clinician practises may also vary widely. Laws dealing with the use of illicit substances vary considerably and penalties may, in some countries, be quite severe. As a result of these differences in the infrastructure for providing mental health care and in legal systems, the first decision a clinician may have to make is whether the traveller's care can be managed at the travel destination or whether the traveller requires repatriation.

While managing mental disorders, health care providers should remain aware of – and ensure protection of, and respect for – the rights of people with mental disorders, in keeping with international covenants and national laws. This should include informing individuals about their rights regarding their treatment, their health condition and treatment options, and obtaining consent for all diagnostic and treatment interventions as appropriate.

Mental disorders are not rare among travellers. Overall, mental health issues are among the leading causes of ill health among travellers, and "psychiatric emergency" is one of the most common medical reasons for air evacuation, along with injury and cardiovascular disease.

10.2 Precautions when undertaking travel

Although some of the events that cause stress cannot be predicted, taking precautions may reduce travel-related stress. Travellers should gather proper information before travel (for example, on the nature of their journey, such as the mode of travel or the journey length, or on the characteristics of their destination and the expected difficulties); this will enable them to maintain their self-confidence and to cope with the unfamiliar. It also allows them to develop strategies to minimize risks. Gathering information before travel helps to reduce the risk of suffering psychological disturbances or aggravating a pre-existing mental disorder.

Neuropsychiatric disturbances (seizures, psychosis and encephalopathy) occur in approximately 1 in 10 000 travellers receiving mefloquine prophylaxis for malaria. Patients with a recent history of neuropsychiatric disorder, including depression, generalized anxiety disorder, or psychotic or seizure disorder, should be prescribed an alternative regimen.

Travellers subject to stress and anxiety, especially concerning air travel, should be helped to develop coping mechanisms. Individuals who are afraid of flying may be referred to specialized courses run by airlines, if available.

Given the potential consequences of a psychiatric emergency arising while travelling overseas, enquiry into psychiatric history or treatment should be a standard part of any pre-travel consultation. Travellers with a significant history of mental disorder should receive specific medical and psychological advice. Those using psychotropic medication should continue the medication while travelling. In certain countries it is a criminal offence to carry a prescription psychotropic medication (for example, benzodiazepine) without proof of prescription. It is thus highly advisable that travellers carry a letter from a physician certifying the need for drugs or other medical items (Chapter 1), or both, as well as documents about their clinical conditions and details about treatment, such as copies of prescriptions. All these documents should be ideally in a language that is understood in the country of travel. Travellers who will be abroad for long periods of time (for example, expatriates or business travellers) can be taught self-monitoring techniques and stress-reduction strategies before departure or during their stay. If drug misuse is suspected, the large variation in the legal status of drug misuse among countries should be emphasized.

If the appropriate precautions are taken, most people affected by a mental disorder whose condition is stable and who are under the supervision of a medical specialist are able to travel abroad.

10.3 Mental disorders

10.3.1 Anxiety disorders

In a study by Matsumoto & Goebert, about 3.5% of all medical in-flight emergencies in the United States were categorized as being caused by mental disorder. In 90% of the in-flight emergencies caused by mental disorder, the diagnosis was an anxiety state, and in only 4% was it a psychotic disorder.

Phobia of flying
Extreme fear of flying may be a symptom of a specific phobia. A specific phobia is an intense, disabling fear of something that poses little or no actual danger. Specific phobias are characterized by marked fear of a specific object or situation or marked avoidance of such objects or situations. In specific phobias, significant emotional distress is caused by these symptoms or avoidance of the situation as well as by the recognition that these feelings or actions are excessive or unreasonable. People with phobia of flying usually dread or avoid flying, and may have anxious anticipation when confronted with vivid descriptions of flights, the need to fly, and the preparations necessary for flying. This fear may severely limit an individual's ability to pursue certain careers or enjoy leisure away from home. Phobia of flying may coexist with other specific phobias. Additionally, anxiolytic medication or alcohol is often used as a means of coping with this fear.

The phobia of flying responds well to exposure-based psychological treatment. Before starting treatment, the individual may need to be educated about aircraft technology and maintenance, control of airspace, or pilot training; worries about these issues may make him or her vulnerable to fears of possible disasters. A typical 2-day treatment regimen focuses exclusively on identifying the anxiety hierarchy and practising desensitization. New virtual-reality technologies that allow therapists to create more realistic environments for desensitization aid this brief approach. However, the equipment to support this approach may be unavailable in most countries. Other techniques that may help passengers to overcome their fear of flying are based on self-control, relaxation and challenging negative thoughts. These techniques may be learned from cognitive behavioural self-help books or from psychotherapists trained in cognitive behavioural therapy.

Panic attacks

Anxiety that is intense enough to occasion an emergency room visit has been noted frequently among psychiatric emergencies occurring in travellers. Panic attacks are characterized by an abrupt onset of intense anxiety with concomitant signs and symptoms of autonomic hyperactivity. Associated feelings of shortness of breath, chest pain, choking, nausea, derealization, and fear of dying may be present. The attack peaks within 10 min, sometimes much more quickly, and may last for 30 min. These attacks may occur as a part of a panic disorder or as a result of substance abuse, such as during cannabis use or alcohol withdrawal. Panic attacks may also occur in those with a phobia of flying. People who experience panic attacks may feel more comfortable in an aisle seat when travelling by plane.

The onset of panic attacks often occurs during or following periods of increasingly stressful life events, and these events may be related to travelling. Since caffeine, certain illicit drugs, and even some over-the-counter cold medications can aggravate the symptoms of anxiety disorders, they should be avoided by people suffering severe anxiety.

10.3.2 Mood disorders and suicide attempts

Depression

The stress of international travel or overseas residence, isolation from family and familiar social support systems, and reactions to a foreign culture and language may all contribute to depression, at least in people who are susceptible. Uncommon but serious problems associated with depression are the risk of suicide or the occurrence of psychotic symptoms, or both.

Depression is characterized by persistent depressed mood or lack of interest occurring over a number of weeks. People who are depressed tend to be relatively inactive, anergic and unmotivated. Associated symptoms may include difficulty sleeping and loss of appetite and weight (occasionally people may sleep or eat more), feelings of worthlessness and hopelessness, suicidal ideation or thoughts of death, poor concentration and memory impairment. Some people may have psychotic features, such as delusions or hallucinations, which are usually consistent with their mood. Depressive episodes may occur as single episodes, as recurrent episodes, or as part of bipolar affective disorder. Treatment, if indicated, should be initiated and monitored by a trained clinician.

Suicide risk

People who are depressed should be assessed in terms of the frequency and persistence of suicidal ideation, their plans for a suicide attempt, whether they have easy access to lethal means for an attempt, the seriousness of their intent, their personal history of suicide attempts (for example, the potential lethality, the chance of discovery), whether there is a family history of suicide or suicide attempts, whether they have psychotic features or are misusing substances, whether they have had major recent adverse life events, and their sociodemographic details (for example, sex, age, and marital and employment status). If the risk of suicide appears to be substantial, immediate hospitalization in a mental health facility (or evacuation to the nearest adequate facility) may be the best option. Hospitalization in non-psychiatric services of general hospitals in order to prevent acts of self-harm is not recommended. However, admission to a general (non-psychiatric) hospital for management of the physical consequences of an act of self-harm may nonetheless be necessary; in such a case, the individual should be closely monitored to prevent subsequent self-harm in the hospital.

Whether or not these options are immediately available, clinicians should try to implement suicide prevention measures; these may include arranging for a 24-hour attendant (a family member, private duty nurse, etc.), and removing any obvious means of suicide (firearms, medications, knives, pesticides, toxic substances, etc.) as long as the individual has thoughts of, or carries out, self-harm. Access to alcohol and other psychoactive substances should be reduced, and an evaluation for withdrawal symptoms should be undertaken. Regular contact is recommended for individuals who volunteer thoughts of self-harm, or who are identified as having planned self-harm in the previous month or performed acts of self-harm in the previous year. Suicidal individuals who exhibit psychotic features or severe problems with substance misuse should be referred to a specialist. It is of note that survivors of suicide attempts may require legal assistance in those countries where attempting suicide is illegal.

Mania

Although relatively uncommon, mania may pose an emergency overseas. The manic state is seen as part of a bipolar affective disorder in which people also have depressive episodes. A manic episode is characterized by an abnormally elevated, euphoric or irritable mood that persists for days or weeks. People with mania frequently present with inflated self-esteem, abundant energy, a decreased need for sleep, heightened libido and negligible insight into the nature of their disorder. These symptoms may lead to poor judgement that affects decisions in various spheres of life (for example, financial, sexual, career, or in terms of substance use). Occasionally, patients develop psychotic symptoms, such as incoherence, delusions and hallucinations. Hypomanic states are less serious versions of mania that usually do not require hospitalization. It is common to find travellers who have initiated a trip because of their elevated mood.

Treatment delivered overseas is frequently aimed at either hospitalization, if possible, or stabilization pending medical evacuation or repatriation. Committing an individual to care under the criterion of posing imminent danger to self or others is not always possible, and the individual's lack of insight may make voluntary consent to treatment difficult to achieve. Frequently, some sort of leverage from family or a sponsoring organization is necessary to obtain the individual's cooperation. Physicians should carry out a medical evaluation that includes assessment and tests for substance misuse (for example, the use of amphetamines or cocaine) since misuse can cause manic symptoms.

10.3.3 Psychotic disorders

A psychotic state is characterized by delusions, hallucinations, thought disorder or severe changes in behaviour (for example, severe self-neglect or catatonia). Psychosis is a state that may occur in many different mental disorders, including mania, depression and many substance use disorders. The presence of psychosis, especially in an individual who is not suffering from a chronic mental disorder, or who has had no prior episodes, represents a psychiatric emergency.

Acute and transient psychotic disorder

Acute and transient psychotic disorder is characterized by rapid onset of symptoms of psychosis and a relatively brief duration (≤ 3 months). Given the known association between stress and acute and transient psychotic disorder, it is not surprising that such disorders have been described in relation to travel stress. It is hypothesized that the isolation of long-distance travel, substance misuse, irregular food and fluid intake, and insomnia may contribute to their occurrence. On the other hand, cultural and individual factors may also be important from the etiological perspective. Some psychotic manifestations may be related to places with historical, artistic or religious significance. A traveller may become overwhelmed at pilgrimage centres such as Mecca, Jerusalem, and Santiago de Compostela, as well as at a variety of holy places in India. In many cases reported from these and other specific sites, the psychotic state evolved rapidly, there was no prior history of such problems, and symptoms resolved quickly with treatment. However, it should be recognized that some people who seemingly develop psychosis in these specific situations might be experiencing an exacerbation or recurrence of pre-existing psychoses, such as schizophrenia.

Management depends upon accurate diagnosis. Since psychotic states may occur as a result of mood disorders, substance use disorders (involving, for example, cannabis), schizophrenia and general medical conditions (for example, cerebral malaria) or medications (for example, mefloquine), these must be excluded. Due attention should be paid to the risk of violence or suicide. If hospitalization and referral to a specialist are not possible, the clinician should use a safe, contained environment that allows for frequent monitoring.

Schizophrenia

Reports of finding travellers with schizophrenia at international airports or at embassies when in need of assistance are by no means rare. Travellers with schizophrenia may be arrested by police for "very strange" or "suspicious" behaviour, and police or family members may contact the embassy. Schizophrenia is characterized by psychotic symptoms that can wax and wane over time. (Symptoms may remit for extended periods, especially with treatment.) Negative symptoms, such as flat affect, lack of motivation, and poverty of thought and speech, are also present for extended periods of time, even in the absence of psychosis. Schizophrenia often begins in the teens or early adulthood. Given the chronic nature of the disorder and the relatively early age of onset, it is unlikely that travel in itself can be considered a causative factor. Individuals with schizophrenia often misuse substances and may have coexisting substance use disorders.

10.3.4 Disorders due to psychoactive substance use

A wide variety of disorders of differing severity are attributable to the use of one or more psychoactive substances. Misuse of all substances is encountered among the population of international travellers. In a study of 1008 young backpackers (aged 18–35 years), Bellis et al. reported that more than half of the sample (55.0%) used at least one illicit drug when backpacking. Individuals showed a significant increase in the frequency of alcohol consumption in the country in which they were travelling compared with their behaviour in their home country. (The proportion of individuals drinking five or more times per week almost doubled, from 20.7% to 40.3%.)

Dependence on psychoactive substances is characterized by craving (a strong desire or compulsion to take the substance); difficulties in controlling substance-taking behaviour (in terms of its onset, termination, or levels of use); physiological withdrawal state (or use of the same or a closely related substance for relieving or avoiding this state) when substance use has ceased or been reduced; tolerance (higher doses of the psychoactive substances are required in order to achieve effects originally produced by lower doses); progressive neglect of alternative pleasures or interests because of the use of the psychoactive substance (more time is necessary to obtain or take the substance or to recover from its effects); and persisting with substance use despite clear evidence of overtly harmful consequences. Travel is unlikely to be a key determinant of the development of substance dependence. However, being in new and sometimes exotic places and freed from the familial and social restraints of home, as well as having easy access to cheap substances, may trigger a relapse in individuals who are in remission.

People with substance dependence who plan to travel sometimes carry small doses of the substances (or a substitute such as methadone) to avoid withdrawal syndrome. Psychoactive substance possession or use is considered a serious crime in quite a few countries. Travellers should be treated for withdrawal and dependence before departure. Travellers who misuse substances may present or be brought to health care professionals abroad because of intoxication or with withdrawal syndromes.

Intoxication

Acute intoxication is a dose-related transient condition that occurs following the administration of alcohol or another psychoactive substance, resulting in disturbances in level of consciousness, thought processes, perception, affect, behaviour, or psychophysiological functions. Almost always, alcohol intoxication (that is, drunkenness) alone does not become a psychiatric emergency, unless the individual becomes violent or suicidal. However, intoxication with stimulants, hallucinogens, phencyclidine, inhalants, and cannabis more commonly result in psychotic states that may present as a psychiatric emergency. Given the complexity of treating these states of intoxication, hospitalization or treatment in an emergency room over the course of hours is preferred over outpatient treatment

Withdrawal

Withdrawal states may also present as psychiatric emergencies. Withdrawal from alcohol or sedatives or hypnotics is usually characterized by autonomic hyperactivity, tremors, insomnia, anxiety and agitation. Occasionally, however, it may be associated with seizures or delirium tremens, a condition marked by delirium, severe autonomic hyperactivity, vivid hallucinations, delusions, severe tremors and agitation. Delirium tremens is associated with significant mortality. People presenting with withdrawal should always be evaluated for concurrent medical conditions and for the use of other substances that might complicate diagnosis or management or diagnosis. Psychosocial support, if available, is helpful for patients undergoing a tapering regime.

Even brief contact with patients following the detection of substance misuse offers the health care professional opportunities to intervene to reduce harm. The individual should be given individualized feedback; advice about reducing or stopping the consumption of substances; and information on how to obtain clean injecting equipment, on safer sexual behaviour, and on risk factors for accidental overdose. They should also be offered the possibility of follow-up. Some people presenting with intoxication, and most people presenting with withdrawal, are likely to be dependent on the substance in question; they should be advised to obtain long-term treatment in their country of origin.

10.4 Other relevant areas of concern

10.4.1 Air rage

Passenger misconduct of an aggressive nature during travel has become a matter of considerable public concern and seems to be increasing in frequency, although it is still not very common. Air rage may vary from verbal threats aimed at crew and fellow passengers to physical assault and other antisocial behaviour. Some physical aggression has been common in air rage but serious injuries have been infrequent. Air rage – like road rage – is predominantly attributed to young males. Although occasional instances may be ascribed to mental disorder, the main factors associated with air rage are alcohol and substance misuse (for example, intoxication or withdrawal), arguments with travel attendants, crowding, delays and lack of information about problems with the journey. Prevention efforts may involve training transport staff.

10.4.2 Culture shock and reverse culture shock

Travel often leads to encounters with new cultures, necessitating adjustment to different customs, lifestyle and languages. Adapting to the new culture is particularly important when travelling for a long period (such as during expatriation or migration). Major cultural change may evoke severe distress in some individuals and is termed "culture shock". This condition arises when individuals suddenly find themselves in a new culture in which they feel completely alien. They may also feel conflict over which aspect of their lifestyle to maintain or change or which new lifestyle to adopt. Children and young adult immigrants often adapt more easily than middle-aged and elderly immigrants because they learn the new language and continue to mature in the new culture. If an individual is part of a family or a group making the transition and the move is positive and planned, stress may be lower. Furthermore, if selected cultural mores can be safely maintained as people integrate into the new culture, then stress will be minimized.

Reactive symptoms are understandable and include anxiety, depression, isolation, fear and a sense of loss of identity during the process of adjustment. Self-understanding, the passage of time, and support from friends, family members and colleagues usually helps to reduce the distress associated with adapting to new cultures and unfamiliar experiences. Distressed individuals who present to health professionals may be helped to understand that experiencing these reactions is natural and that distress will subside as they adapt to the new culture. Joining activities in the new community and actively trying to meet neighbours and co-workers may lessen culture shock.

Returning home may also be a psychological challenge for people who have been travelling and living abroad for a prolonged period of time, especially if overseas travel has been particularly enjoyable or if their future life is expected to be less exciting and fulfilling. Some younger or long-term travellers may exhibit a strong desire to remain within the new culture and a dread of returning home. In others, a sense of loss and bereavement may set in after the return, when travellers and their relatives realize that things have changed and that they have grown further apart as a result of their differing experiences. This may lead to feelings of surprise, frustration, confusion, anxiety and sadness – often termed reverse culture shock. Sometimes friends and relatives may themselves be hurt and surprised by the reaction of those who have returned. Self-understanding and the ability to explain the situation may help all parties to restore healthy reactions and relationships.

Further reading

Bellis MA et al. Effects of backpacking holidays in Australia on alcohol, tobacco and drug use of UK residents. *BMC Public Health*, 2007, 7:1 (available at http://www.biomedcentral.com/content/pdf/1471-2458-7-1.pdf).

Committee to Advise on Tropical Medicine and Travel (CATMAT). Travel statement on jet lag. *Canada Communicable Disease Report*, 2003, 29:4–8.

Gordon H, Kingham M, Goodwin T. Air travel by passengers with mental disorder. *Psychiatric Bulletin*, 2004, 28:295–297.

Lavernhe JP, Ivanoff S. Medical assistance to travellers: a new concept in insurance – cooperation with an airline. *Aviation Space and Environmental Medicine*, 1985, 56:367–370.

Matsumoto K, Goebert D. In-flight psychiatric emergencies. *Aviation Space and Environmental Medicine*, 2001, 72:919–923.

Sanford C. Urban medicine: threats to health of travellers to developing world cities. *Journal of Travel Medicine*, 2004, 11:313–327.

Sugden R. Fear of flying – Aviophobia. In: Keystone JS et al., eds. *Travel medicine*. Edinburgh, Mosby, 2004: 361–365.

Tourism highlights: 2007 edition. Madrid, World Tourism Organization, 2007.

Tran TM, Browning J, Dell ML. Psychosis with paranoid delusions after a therapeutic dose of mefloquine: a case report. *Malaria Journal*, 2006, 5:74.

Valk TH. Psychiatric disorders and psychiatric emergencies overseas. In: Keystone JS et al., eds. *Travel medicine*. Edinburgh, Mosby, 2004: 367–377.

Waterhouse J et al. Jet lag: trends and coping strategies. *Lancet*, 2007, 369:1117–1129.

Country list[1]
Yellow fever vaccination requirements and recommendations; and malaria situation

Introduction

The information provided for each country includes the country's stated requirements for yellow fever vaccination, WHO recommendation for travellers regarding yellow fever vaccinations, and details concerning the malaria situation and recommended prevention of the disease.[2,3]

Yellow fever

Yellow fever vaccination

Yellow fever vaccination is carried out for two different purposes:

1. To prevent the international spread of the disease by protecting countries from the risk of importing or spreading the yellow fever virus. These are requirements established by the country.

The countries that require proof of vaccination[2] are those where the disease may or may not occur and where the mosquito vector and potential non-human primate hosts of yellow fever are present. Any importation of the virus into such countries by infected travellers could result in its propagation and establishment, leading to a permanent risk of infection for the human population. Proof of vaccination is often required for travellers arriving from countries with risk of yellow fever transmission and sometimes for travellers in transit through such countries. A

---

[1] For the purpose of this publication, the terms "country" and "countries" cover countries, territories and areas.

[2] Please note that the requirements for vaccination of infants over 6 months of age by some countries are not in accordance with WHO's advice (Chapter 6). Travellers should, however, be informed that the requirement exists for entry into the countries concerned.

[3] WHO publishes these requirements for informational purposes only; this publication does not constitute an endorsement or confirmation that such requirements are in accordance with the provisions of the International Health Regulations.

meeting of yellow fever experts organized in 2010 proposed that under 12 h of airport transit the risk of yellow fever is almost non-existent and therefore that a proof of vaccination might not be necessary. This information is being provided to WHO Member States, but travellers are recommended to consult individual country requirements by contacting the embassy(ies) of the country(ies) they intend to visit. It should be noted that some countries require proof of vaccination from all travellers.

Countries requiring yellow fever vaccination for entry do so in accordance with the International Health Regulations. Country requirements are subject to change at any time. Updates can be found at: http://www.who.int/ith. This chapter contains information on yellow fever requirements as provided by countries.

The fact that a country has no requirement for yellow fever vaccination does not imply that there is no risk of yellow fever transmission.

2. To protect individual travellers who may be exposed to yellow fever infection.

The risk of yellow fever transmission depends on the presence of the virus in the country in humans, mosquitoes or animals. As yellow fever is frequently fatal for those who have not been vaccinated, vaccination is recommended for all travellers (with few exceptions, Chapter 6) visiting areas where there is a risk of yellow fever transmission.

WHO determines those areas where "a risk of yellow fever transmission is present" on the basis of the diagnosis of cases of yellow fever in humans and/or animals, the results of yellow fever sero-surveys and the presence of vectors and animal reservoirs.[4]

In consultation with experts, WHO has revised the criteria for the risk of yellow fever transmission. Updates have been made for Argentina, Bolivarian Republic of Venezuela, Brazil, Colombia, the Democratic Republic of the Congo, Ecuador, Eritrea, Ethiopia, Kenya, Panama, Paraguay, Peru, Sao Tome and Principe, Somalia, Trinidad and Tobago, United Republic of Tanzania and Zambia (Country list below, Annex 1 and yellow fever map).

Decisions regarding the use of yellow fever vaccine for travellers must weigh several factors, including the risk of travel-associated yellow fever virus disease, country

---

[4] More extensive descriptions of the classifications that define areas with risk of yellow fever virus transmission can be found at http://www.who.int/ith/YFrisk.pdf. These classifications inform the vaccine recommendations listed here.

requirements, and the potential for serious adverse events following yellow fever vaccination (Chapter 6).

The table below summarizes WHO's revised recommendations for yellow fever vaccination for travellers.

Yellow fever vaccination category	Rationale for recommendation
Recommended	Yellow fever vaccination is recommended for all travellers ≥9 months old in areas where there is evidence of persistent or periodic yellow fever virus transmission.
Generally not recommended	Yellow fever vaccination is *generally not recommended* in areas where there is low potential for yellow fever virus exposure (no human yellow fever cases ever reported and evidence to suggest only low levels of yellow fever virus transmission in the past). However, vaccination might be considered for a small subset of travellers to these areas, who are at increased risk of exposure to mosquitoes or unable to avoid mosquito bites. When considering vaccination, any traveller must take into account the risk of being infected with yellow fever virus, country entry requirements, as well as individual risk factors (e.g. age, immune status) for serious vaccine-associated adverse events.

Annex 1 provides a summary list of countries with risk of yellow fever transmission in whole or in part, as well as a list of countries that require proof of yellow fever vaccination as a condition for entry.

Other diseases

Cholera. No country reports a requirement for a certificate of vaccination against cholera as a condition for entry. For information on selective use of cholera vaccines, Chapter 6.

Smallpox. Since the global eradication of smallpox was certified in 1980, WHO does not recommend smallpox vaccination for travellers.

Other infectious diseases. Information on the main infectious disease threats for travellers, their geographical distribution, and corresponding precautions are provided in Chapter 5. Chapter 6 provides information on vaccine-preventable diseases.

Malaria

General information about malaria, its geographical distribution and details of preventive measures are included in Chapter 7. Protective measures against mosquito bites are described in Chapter 3. Specific information for each country is provided in this section, including epidemiological details for all countries with malarious areas (geographical and seasonal distribution, altitude, predominant species, reported resistance). The recommended prevention is also indicated. For each country, recommended prevention is decided on the basis of the following factors: the risk of contracting malaria; the prevailing species of malaria parasites in the area; the level and spread of drug resistance reported from the country; and the possible risk of serious side-effects resulting from the use of the various prophylactic drugs. Where *Plasmodium falciparum* and *P. vivax* both occur, prevention of falciparum malaria takes priority. Unless the malaria risk is defined as due "exclusively" to a certain species (*P. falciparum* or *P. vivax*), travellers may be at risk of any of the parasite species, including mixed infections.

The numbers I, II, III and IV refer to the type of prevention based on the table below.

	Malaria risk	Type of prevention
Type I	Very limited risk of malaria transmission	Mosquito bite prevention only
Type II	Risk of *P. vivax* malaria only; or fully chloroquine-sensitive *P. falciparum*	Mosquito bite prevention plus chloroquine chemoprophylaxis
Type III[a]	Risk of *P. vivax* and *P. falciparum* malaria transmission, combined with emerging chloroquine resistance	Mosquito bite prevention plus chloroquine+proguanil chemoprophylaxis
Type IV	(1) High risk of *P. falciparum* malaria, combined with reported antimalarial drug resistance; or (2) Moderate/low risk of *P. falciparum* malaria, combined with reported high levels of drug resistance[b]	Mosquito bite prevention plus atovaquone–proguanil, doxycycline or mefloquine chemoprophylaxis (select according to reported resistance pattern)

[a] The areas where Type III prevention is still an option are parts of Colombia and India, Nepal, Sri Lanka and Tajikistan. If needed, Type IV prevention can be used instead.

[b] Alternatively, when travelling to rural areas with multidrug-resistant malaria and only a very low risk of *P. falciparum* infection, mosquito bite prevention can be combined with stand-by emergency treatment.

203

AFGHANISTAN

Yellow fever

Country requirement: a yellow fever vaccination certificate is required from travellers arriving from countries with risk of yellow fever transmission.

Yellow fever vaccine recommendation: no

Malaria: Malaria risk – *P. falciparum* and *P. vivax* – exists from May to November inclusive below 2000 m. *P. falciparum* resistant to chloroquine and sulfadoxine–pyrimethamine reported.

Recommended prevention in risk areas: **IV**

ALBANIA

Yellow fever

Country requirement: a yellow fever vaccination certificate is required from travellers over 1 year of age arriving from countries with risk of yellow fever transmission.

Yellow fever vaccine recommendation: no

ALGERIA

Yellow fever

Country requirement: a yellow fever vaccination certificate is required from travellers over 1 year of age arriving from countries with risk of yellow fever transmission.

Yellow fever vaccine recommendation: no

Malaria: Malaria risk is limited. Small foci of local transmission (*P. vivax*) have previously been reported in the six southern and south-eastern wilayas (Adrar, El Oued, Ghardaia, Illizi, Ouargla, Tamanrasset), with isolated local *P. falciparum* transmission reported from the two southernmost wilayas in areas under the influence of trans-Saharan migration. Three locally acquired cases were reported in 2008.

Recommended prevention in risk areas: **I**

AMERICAN SAMOA

Yellow fever

Country requirement: no

Yellow fever vaccine recommendation: no

ANDORRA

Yellow fever

Country requirement: no

Yellow fever vaccine recommendation: no

ANGOLA

Yellow fever

Country requirement: a yellow fever vaccination certificate is required from all travellers over 1 year of age.

Yellow fever vaccine recommendation: yes

Malaria: Malaria risk due predominantly to *P. falciparum* exists throughout the year in the whole country. Resistance to chloroquine and sulfadoxine–pyrimethamine reported.

Recommended prevention: **IV**

ANGUILLA

Yellow fever

Country requirement: a yellow fever vaccination certificate is required from travellers over 1 year of age arriving from countries with risk of yellow fever transmission.

Yellow fever vaccine recommendation: no

ANTIGUA AND BARBUDA

Yellow fever

Country requirement: a yellow fever vaccination certificate is required from travellers over 1 year of age arriving from countries with risk of yellow fever transmission.

Yellow fever vaccine recommendation: no

ARGENTINA

Yellow fever

Country requirement: no

Yellow fever vaccine recommendation: yes

Recommended for all travellers aged 9 months and over going to northern and north-eastern forested areas of Argentina bordering Brazil and Paraguay where altitudes are <2300 m (Map). Travellers to departments in the following provinces should be vaccinated: Misiones (all departments) and Corrientes (Berón de Astrada, Capital, General Alvear, General Paz, Ituzaingó, Itatí, Paso de los Libres, San Cosme, San Martín, San Miguel, Santo Tomé). Vaccination is also recommended for travellers visiting Iguazu Falls.

Generally not recommended[1] for travellers whose itineraries are limited to the designated depart-

[1] Yellow fever vaccination is *generally not recommended* in areas where there is low potential for exposure to yellow fever virus. However, vaccination might be considered for a small subset of travellers to these areas, who are at increased risk of exposure to yellow fever virus (e.g. prolonged travel, extensive exposure to mosquitoes, inability to avoid mosquito bites). When considering vaccination, any traveller must take into account the risk of being infected with yellow fever virus, country entry requirements, as well as individual risk factors (e.g. age, immune status) for serious vaccine-associated adverse events.

ments in the following provinces, where altitudes are <2300 m: Formosa (all departments), Chaco (Bermejo) Jujuy (Ledesma, San Pedro, Santa Bárbara, Valle Grande), and Salta (Anta, General José de San Martín, Oran, Rivadavia) (Map).

Not recommended for travellers whose itineraries are limited to areas at altitudes >2300 m and all provinces and departments not listed above.

Malaria: Malaria risk due exclusively to *P. vivax* is very low and is confined to rural areas along the borders with Plurinational State of Bolivia (lowlands of Salta province) and with Paraguay (lowlands of Chaco and Misiones provinces).

Recommended prevention in risk areas: **II**

ARMENIA
Yellow fever

Country requirement: no

Yellow fever vaccine recommendation: no

Malaria: Limited malaria risk due exclusively to *P. vivax* may exist focally from June to October inclusive in some villages located in Ararat Valley. No risk in tourist areas. No indigenous cases reported since 2006.

Recommended prevention in risk areas: **I**

AUSTRALIA
Yellow fever

Country requirement: a yellow fever vaccination certificate is required from travellers over 1 year of age entering Australia within 6 days of having stayed overnight or longer in a country with risk of yellow fever transmission, excluding Galapagos Islands in Ecuador and limited to Misiones province in Argentina, but including Sao Toe and Principe, Somalia and the United Republic of Tanzania.

Yellow fever vaccine recommendation: no

AUSTRIA
Yellow fever

Country requirement: no

Yellow fever vaccine recommendation: no

AZERBAIJAN
Yellow fever

Country requirement: no

Yellow fever vaccine recommendation: no

Malaria: Malaria risk due exclusively to *P. vivax* exists from June to October inclusive in lowland areas, mainly in the area between the Kura and Arax rivers.

Recommended prevention in risk areas: **II**

AZORES see PORTUGAL

BAHAMAS
Yellow fever

Country requirement: a yellow fever vaccination certificate is required from travellers over 1 year of age arriving from countries with risk of yellow fever transmission.

Yellow fever vaccine recommendation: no

Malaria: Sporadic local transmission of *P. falciparum* has been reported in recent years on Great Exuma island only, subsequent to international importation of parasites. No risk on other islands.

Recommended prevention on Great Exuma: **I**

BAHRAIN
Yellow fever

Country requirement: a yellow fever vaccination certificate is required from travellers over 1 year of age arriving from countries with risk of yellow fever transmission.

Yellow fever vaccine recommendation: no

BANGLADESH
Yellow fever

Country requirement: a yellow fever vaccination certificate is required from travellers over 1 year of age arriving from countries with risk of yellow fever transmission.

Yellow fever vaccine recommendation: no

Malaria: Malaria risk exists throughout the year in the whole country excluding Dhaka city, with highest risk in Chittagong Division, the districts of Mymensingh, Netrakona and Sherpur in Dhaka Division, and Kurigram district in Rajshahi Division. *P. falciparum* resistant to chloroquine and sulfadoxine–pyrimethamine reported.

Recommended prevention in risk areas: **IV**

BARBADOS

Yellow fever

Country requirement: a yellow fever vaccination certificate is required from travellers over 1 year of age arriving from countries with risk of yellow fever transmission except Guyana and Trinidad and Tobago.

Yellow fever vaccine recommendation: no

BELARUS

Yellow fever

Country requirement: no

Yellow fever vaccine recommendation: no

BELGIUM

Yellow fever

Country requirement: no

Yellow fever vaccine recommendation: no

BELIZE

Yellow fever

Country requirement: a yellow fever vaccination certificate is required from travellers over 1 year of age arriving from countries with risk of yellow fever transmission.

Yellow fever vaccine recommendation: no

Malaria: Malaria risk due predominantly to *P. vivax* exists in all districts but varies within regions. Risk is moderate in Stan Creek and Toledo Districts; and low in Cayo, Corozal and Orange Walk.

Recommended prevention in risk areas: **II**

BENIN

Yellow fever

Country requirement: a yellow fever vaccination certificate is required from all travellers over 1 year of age.

Yellow fever vaccine recommendation: yes

Malaria: Malaria risk due predominantly to *P. falciparum* exists throughout the year in the whole country. Resistance to chloroquine and sulfadoxine–pyrimethamine reported.

Recommended prevention: **IV**

BERMUDA

Yellow fever

Country requirement: no

Yellow fever vaccine recommendation: no

BHUTAN

Yellow fever

Country requirement: a yellow fever vaccination certificate is required from travellers arriving from countries with risk of yellow fever transmission.

Yellow fever vaccine recommendation: no

Malaria: Malaria risk exists throughout the year in the southern belt of the country comprising five districts: Chhukha, Geyleg-phug, Samchi, Samdrup Jonkhar and Shemgang. *P. falciparum* resistant to chloroquine and sulfadoxine–pyrimethamine reported.

Recommended prevention in risk areas: **IV**

BOLIVIA (PLURINATIONAL STATE OF)

Yellow fever

Country requirement: a yellow fever vaccination certificate is required from travellers over 1 year of age arriving from countries with risk of yellow fever transmission.

Yellow fever vaccine recommendation: yes

Recommended for all travellers aged 9 months of age and over travelling to the following area east of the Andes at altitudes below 2300 m: the entire departments of Beni, Pando, and Santa Cruz, and designated areas (Map) of Chuquisaca, Cochabamba, La Paz and Tarija.

Not recommended for travellers whose itineraries are limited to areas at altitudes above 2300 m and all areas not listed above, including the cities of La Paz and Sucre.

Malaria: Malaria risk due predominantly (94%) to *P. vivax* exists throughout the year in the whole country below 2500 m. Falciparum malaria occurs in Santa Cruz and in the northern departments of Beni and Pando, especially in the localities of Guayaramerín and Riberalta. *P. falciparum* resistant to chloroquine and sulfadoxine–pyrimethamine reported.

Recommended prevention in risk areas: **II**; in Beni, Pando and Santa Cruz: **IV**

BOSNIA AND HERZEGOVINA

Yellow fever

Country requirement: no

Yellow fever vaccine recommendation: no

BOTSWANA

Yellow fever

Country requirement: a yellow fever vaccination certificate is required from travellers over 1 year of age arriving from or having passed through countries with risk of yellow fever transmission.

Yellow fever vaccine recommendation: no

Malaria: Malaria risk due predominantly to *P. falciparum* exists from November to May/June in the northern parts of the country: Boteti, Chobe, Ngamiland, Okavango, Tutume districts/sub-districts. Chloroquine-resistant *P. falciparum* reported.

Recommended prevention in risk areas: **IV**

BRAZIL

Yellow fever

Country requirement: no

Yellow fever vaccine recommendation: yes

Recommended for all travellers aged 9 months or over going to the following areas: the entire states of Acre, Amapá, Amazones, Distrito Federal (including the capital city of Brasília), Goiás, Maranhão, Mato Grosso, Mato Grosso do Sul, Minas Gerais, Pará, Rondônia, Roraima and Tocantins, and designated areas (Map) of the following states: Bahia, Paraná, Piauí, Rio Grande do Sul, Santa Catarina and São Paulo. Vaccination is also recommended for travellers visiting Iguazu Falls.

Not recommended for travellers whose itineraries are limited to areas not listed above, including the cities of Fortaleza, Recife, Rio de Janeiro, Salvador and São Paulo (Map).

Malaria: In the states outside "Legal Amazonia", the risk of malaria transmission is negligible or non-existent. Malaria risk – *P. vivax* (84%), *P. falciparum* (15%), mixed infections (1%) – is present in most forested areas below 900 m within the nine states of the "Legal Amazonia" region (Acre, Amapá, Amazonas, Maranhão (western part), Mato Grosso (northern part), Pará (except Belém City), Rondônia, Roraima and Tocantins (western part)). Transmission intensity varies from one municipality to another, and is higher in jungle mining areas, in agricultural settlements less than 5 years old, and in some peripheral urban areas of Cruzeiro do Sul, Manaus and Pôrto Velho. Malaria also occurs on the periphery of large cities such as Boa Vista, Macapá, Maraba, Rio Branco and Santarém. Multidrug resistant *P. falciparum* reported. *P. vivax* resistance to chloroquine reported.

Recommended prevention in risk areas: **IV**

BRITISH VIRGIN ISLANDS

Yellow fever

Country requirement: no

Yellow fever vaccine recommendation: no

BRUNEI DARUSSALAM

Yellow fever

Country requirement: a yellow fever vaccination certificate is required from travellers over 1 year of age arriving from countries with risk of yellow fever transmission or having passed through areas partly or wholly at risk of yellow fever transmission within the preceding 6 days.

Yellow fever vaccine recommendation: no

Malaria: Human *P. knowlesi* infection reported.

Recommended prevention: **mosquito bite prevention only**

BULGARIA

Yellow fever

Country requirement: no

Yellow fever vaccine recommendation: no

BURKINA FASO

Yellow fever

Country requirement: a yellow fever vaccination certificate is required from all travellers over 1 year of age.

Yellow fever vaccine recommendation: yes

Malaria: Malaria risk due predominantly to *P. falciparum* exists throughout the year in the whole country. Resistance to chloroquine and sulfadoxine–pyrimethamine reported.

Recommended prevention: **IV**

BURMA see MYANMAR

BURUNDI

Yellow fever

Country requirement: a yellow fever vaccination certificate is required from all travellers over 1 year of age.

Yellow fever vaccine recommendation: yes

Malaria: Malaria risk due predominantly to *P. falciparum* exists throughout the year in the whole country. Resistance to chloroquine and sulfadoxine–pyrimethamine reported.

Recommended prevention: **IV**

207

CAMBODIA

Yellow fever

Country requirement: a yellow fever vaccination certificate is required from travellers over 1 year of age arriving from countries with risk of yellow fever transmission.

Yellow fever vaccine recommendation: no

Malaria: Malaria risk due predominantly to *P. falciparum* exists throughout the year in the whole country except in Phnom Penh and close to Tonle Sap. Risk within the tourist area of Angkor Wat is negligible. *P. falciparum* resistant to chloroquine and sulfadoxine–pyrimethamine reported. Resistance to mefloquine and resistance to artesunate reported in south-western provinces.

Recommended prevention in risk areas: **IV**

CAMEROON

Yellow fever

Country requirement: a yellow fever vaccination certificate is required from all travellers over 1 year of age.

Yellow fever vaccine recommendation: yes

Malaria: Malaria risk due predominantly to *P. falciparum* exists throughout the year in the whole country. Resistance to chloroquine and sulfadoxine–pyrimethamine reported.

Recommended prevention: **IV**

CANADA

Yellow fever

Country requirement: no

Yellow fever vaccine recommendation: no

CANARY ISLANDS *see* SPAIN

CAPE VERDE

Yellow fever

Country requirement: a yellow fever vaccination certificate is required from travellers over 1 year of age arriving from countries with risk of yellow fever transmission.

Yellow fever vaccine recommendation: no

Malaria: Limited malaria risk due predominantly to *P. falciparum* exists from August to November inclusive in Santiago island (35 locally acquired

cases reported in 2009), and in Boavista island (10 locally acquired cases reported in 2009).

Recommended prevention in risk areas: **I**

CAYMAN ISLANDS

Yellow fever

Country requirement: no

Yellow fever vaccine recommendation: no

CENTRAL AFRICAN REPUBLIC

Yellow fever

Country requirement: a yellow fever vaccination certificate is required from all travellers over 1 year of age.

Yellow fever vaccine recommendation: yes

Malaria: Malaria risk due predominantly to *P. falciparum* exists throughout the year in the whole country. Resistance to chloroquine and sulfadoxine–pyrimethamine reported.

Recommended prevention: **IV**

CHAD

Yellow fever

Country requirement: a yellow fever vaccination certificate is required from travellers arriving from countries with risk of yellow fever transmission.

Yellow fever vaccine recommendation: yes

Recommended for all travellers aged 9 months or over travelling to areas south of the Sahara Desert (Map).

Not recommended for travellers whose itineraries are limited to areas within the Sahara Desert (Map).

Malaria: Malaria risk due predominantly to *P. falciparum* exists throughout the year in the whole country. Resistance to chloroquine and sulfadoxine–pyrimethamine reported.

Recommended prevention: **IV**

CHILE

Yellow fever

Country requirement: no

Yellow fever vaccine recommendation: no

CHINA

Yellow fever

Country requirement: a yellow fever vaccination certificate is required from travellers over 9 months

of age arriving from countries with risk of yellow fever transmission.

Yellow fever vaccine recommendation: no

Malaria: Malaria risk, including *P. falciparum* malaria, exists in Yunnan and to a lesser extent in Hainan. *P. falciparum* resistance to chloroquine and sulfadoxine-pyrimethamine reported. Limited risk of *P. vivax* malaria exists in southern and some central provinces, including Anhui, Guizhou, Henan, Hubei, Jiangsu. There is no malaria risk in urban areas.

Recommended prevention in risk areas: **II**; in Hainan and Yunnan, **IV**

CHINA, HONG KONG SAR

Yellow fever

Country requirement: no

Yellow fever vaccine recommendation: no

CHINA, MACAO SAR

Yellow fever

Country requirement: no

Yellow fever vaccine recommendation: no

CHRISTMAS ISLAND

(Indian Ocean)

Yellow fever

Same requirements as mainland Australia.

Yellow fever vaccine recommendation: no

COLOMBIA

Yellow fever

Country requirement: no

Yellow fever vaccination recommendation: yes

Recommended for all travellers aged 9 months or over travelling to the following departments at altitudes below 2300 m (Map): Amazonas, Antioquia, Arauca, Atlántico, Bolivar, Boyacá, Caldas, Caquetá, Casanare, Cauca, Cesar, Córdoba, Cundinamarca, Guainía, Guaviare, Huila, Magdalena, Meta, Norte de Santander, Putumayo, Quindio, Risaralda, San Andrés and Providencia, Santander, Sucre, Tolima, Vaupés, Vichada, Choco (only the municipalities of Acandí, Juradó, Riosucio, and Unguía), and La Guajira (only the municipalities of Albania, Barrancas, Dibulla, Distracción, El Molino, Fonseca, Hatonuevo, La Jagua del Pilar, Maicao, Manaure, Riohacha, San Juan del Cesar, Urumita, and Villanueva).

Generally not recommended[1] for travellers whose itineraries are limited to the following areas west of the Andes at altitudes below 2300 m: the departments of Cauca, Nariño and Valle de Cauca, central and southern Choco, and the cities of Barranquilla, Cali, Cartagena and Medellín (Map).

Not recommended for travellers whose itineraries are limited to all areas above 2300 m, including the city of Bogotá and the municipality of Uribia in La Guajira department.

Malaria: Malaria risk – *P. vivax* (72%), *P. falciparum* (27%) – is high throughout the year in rural/jungle areas below 1600 m, especially in municipalities of the regions of Amazonia, Orinoquía, Pacífico and Urabá Bajo Cauca. Transmission intensity varies by department, with the highest risk in Amazonas, Antioquia, Chocó, Córdoba, Guaviare, La Guajira, Nariño and Vichada. Chloroquine-resistant *P. falciparum* exists in Amazonia, Pacífico and Urabá-Bajo Cauca. Resistance to sulfadoxine-pyrimethamine reported.

Recommended prevention in risk areas: **III**; in Amazonia, Pacífico and Urabá-Bajo Cauca: **IV**

COMOROS

Yellow fever

Country requirement: no

Yellow fever vaccine recommendation: no

Malaria: Malaria risk due predominantly to *P. falciparum* exists throughout the year in the whole country. Resistance to chloroquine and sulfadoxine-pyrimethamine reported.

Recommended prevention: **IV**

CONGO

Yellow fever

Country requirement: a yellow fever vaccination certificate is required from all travellers over 1 year of age.

Yellow fever vaccine recommendation: yes

---

[1] Yellow fever vaccination is *generally not recommended* in areas where there is low potential for exposure to yellow fever virus. However, vaccination might be considered for a small subset of travellers to these areas, who are at increased risk of exposure to yellow fever virus (e.g. prolonged travel, extensive exposure to mosquitoes, inability to avoid mosquito bites). When considering vaccination, any traveller must take into account the risk of being infected with yellow fever virus, country entry requirements, as well as individual risk factors (e.g. age, immune status) for serious vaccine-associated adverse events.

Malaria: Malaria risk due predominantly to *P. falciparum* exists throughout the year in the whole country. Resistance to chloroquine and sulfadoxine–pyrimethamine reported.

Recommended prevention: **IV**

COOK ISLANDS
Yellow fever

Country requirement: no

Yellow fever vaccine recommendation: no

COSTA RICA
Yellow fever

Country requirement: a yellow fever vaccination certificate is required from travellers ove 9 months of age arriving from countries with risk of yellow fever transmission with the exception of Argentina, Panama and Trinidad and Tobago

Yellow fever vaccine recommendation: no

Malaria: Malaria risk due almost exclusively to *P. vivax* occurs throughout the year in the province of Limón, mostly in the canton of Matina. Negligible or no risk of malaria transmission exists in the other cantons of the country.

Recommended prevention in risk areas: **II**

CÔTE D'IVOIRE
Yellow fever

Country requirement: a yellow fever vaccination certificate is required from travellers over 1 year of age.

Yellow fever vaccine recommendation: yes

Malaria: Malaria risk due predominantly to *P. falciparum* exists throughout the year in the whole country. Resistance to chloroquine and sulfadoxine–pyrimethamine reported.

Recommended prevention: **IV**

CROATIA
Yellow fever

Country requirement: no

Yellow fever vaccine recommendation: no

CUBA
Yellow fever

Country requirement: no

Yellow fever vaccine recommendation: no

CYPRUS
Yellow fever

Country requirement: no

Yellow fever vaccine recommendation: no

CZECH REPUBLIC
Yellow fever

Country requirement: no

Yellow fever vaccine recommendation: no

DEMOCRATIC PEOPLE'S REPUBLIC OF KOREA
Yellow fever

Country requirement: a yellow fever vaccination certificate is required from travellers over 1 year of age arriving from countries with risk of yellow fever transmission.

Yellow fever vaccine recommendation: no

Malaria: Limited malaria risk due exclusively to *P. vivax* exists in some southern areas.

Recommended prevention in risk areas: **I**

DEMOCRATIC REPUBLIC OF THE CONGO (FORMERLY ZAIRE)
Yellow fever

Country requirement: a yellow fever vaccination certificate is required from all travellers over 1 year of age.

Yellow fever vaccine recommendation: yes

Recommended for all travellers aged 9 months or over, except as mentioned below.

Generally not recommended[1] for travellers whose itineraries are limited to Katanga Province.

Malaria: Malaria risk due predominantly to *P. falciparum* exists throughout the year in the whole country. Resistance to chloroquine and sulfadoxine–pyrimethamine reported.

Recommended prevention: **IV**

---

[1] Yellow fever vaccination is *generally not recommended* in areas where there is low potential for exposure to yellow fever virus. However, vaccination might be considered for a small subset of travellers to these areas, who are at increased risk of exposure to yellow fever virus (e.g. prolonged travel, extensive exposure to mosquitoes, inability to avoid mosquito bites). When considering vaccination, any traveller must take into account the risk of being infected with yellow fever virus, country entry requirements, as well as individual risk factors (e.g. age, immune status) for serious vaccine-associated adverse events.

DENMARK

Yellow fever

Country requirement: no

Yellow fever vaccine recommendation: no

DJIBOUTI

Yellow fever

Country requirement: a yellow fever vaccination certificate is required from travellers over 1 year of age arriving from countries with risk of yellow fever transmission.

Yellow fever vaccine recommendation: no

Malaria: Malaria risk due predominantly to *P. falciparum* exists throughout the year in the whole country. Resistance to chloroquine and sulfadoxine–pyrimethamine reported.

Recommended prevention: **IV**

DOMINICA

Yellow fever

Country requirement: a yellow fever vaccination certificate is required from travellers over 1 year of age arriving from countries with risk of yellow fever transmission.

Yellow fever vaccine recommendation: no

DOMINICAN REPUBLIC

Yellow fever

Country requirement: no

Yellow fever vaccine recommendation: no

Malaria: Malaria risk due exclusively to *P. falciparum* exists throughout the year, especially in the western provinces of Dajabón, Elias Pina and San Juan. Risk in other areas is low to negligible. There is no evidence of *P. falciparum* resistance to any antimalarial drug.

Recommended prevention in risk areas: **II**

ECUADOR

Yellow fever

Country requirement: a yellow fever vaccination certificate is required from travellers over 1 year of age arriving from countries with risk of yellow fever transmission. Nationals and residents of Ecuador are required to possess certificates of vaccination on their departure to an area with risk of yellow fever transmission.

Yellow fever vaccine recommendation: yes

Recommended for all travellers aged 9 months or over travelling to the following provinces east of the Andes at altitudes below 2300 m: Morona-Santiago, Napo, Orellana, Pastaza, Sucumbios and Zamora-Chinchipe (Map).

Generally not recommended[1] for travellers whose itineraries are limited to the following provinces west of the Andes and at altitudes below 2300 m: Esmeraldas, Guayas, Los Rios and Manabi, and designated areas of Azuay, Bolivar, Canar, Carchi, Chimborazo, Cotopaxi, El Oro, Imbabura, Loja, Pichincha and Tungurahua (Map).

Not recommended for travellers whose itineraries are limited to all areas above 2300 m altitude, the cities of Guayaquil and Quito, and the Galápagos Islands (Map).

Malaria: Malaria risk – *P. vivax* (87%), *P. falciparum* (13%) – exists throughout the year below 1500 m, with moderate transmission risk in coastal provinces. There is no risk in Guayaquil, Quito and other cities of the Inter-Andean region. *P. falciparum* resistance to chloroquine and sulfadoxine–pyrimethamine reported.

Recommended prevention in risk areas: **IV**

EGYPT

Yellow fever

Country requirement: a yellow fever vaccination certificate is required from travellers over 1 year of age arriving from countries with risk of yellow fever transmission.

All arrivals from Sudan are required to possess either a vaccination certificate or a location certificate issued by a Sudanese official centre stating that they have not been in Sudan south of 15°N within the previous 6 days.

Yellow fever vaccine recommendation: no

Malaria: Very limited *P. falciparum* and *P. vivax* malaria risk may exist from June to October inclusive in El Faiyûm governorate (no indigenous cases reported since 1998).

Recommended prevention: **none**

---

[1] Yellow fever vaccination is *generally not recommended* in areas where there is low potential for exposure to yellow fever virus. However, vaccination might be considered for a small subset of travellers to these areas, who are at increased risk of exposure to yellow fever virus (e.g. prolonged travel, extensive exposure to mosquitoes, inability to avoid mosquito bites). When considering vaccination, any traveller must take into account the risk of being infected with yellow fever virus, country entry requirements, as well as individual risk factors (e.g. age, immune status) for serious vaccine-associated adverse events.

EL SALVADOR

Yellow fever

Country requirement: a yellow fever vaccination certificate is required from travellers over 1 year of age arriving from countries with risk of yellow fever transmission.

Yellow fever vaccine recommendation: no

Malaria: Very low malaria risk due almost exclusively to *P. vivax* exists in rural areas of migratory influence from Guatemala. Sporadic vivax malaria cases are reported from other parts of the country.

Recommended prevention in risk areas: **I**

EQUATORIAL GUINEA

Yellow fever

Country requirement: a yellow fever vaccination certificate is required from travellers arriving from countries with risk of yellow fever transmission.

Yellow fever vaccine recommendation: yes

Malaria: Malaria risk due predominantly to *P. falciparum* exists throughout the year in the whole country. Resistance to chloroquine and sulfadoxine–pyrimethamine reported.

Recommended prevention: **IV**

ERITREA

Yellow fever

Country requirement: a yellow fever vaccination certificate is required from travellers arriving from countries with risk of yellow fever transmission.

Yellow fever vaccine recommendation: in general, no

Generally not recommended[1] for travellers going to the following states: Anseba, Debub, Gash Barka, Mae Kel and Semenawi Keih Bahri.

Not recommended for all other areas not listed above, including the islands of the Dahlak Archipelagos (Map).

Malaria: Malaria risk – *P. falciparum* and *P. vivax* – exists throughout the year in the whole coun-

try below 2200 m. There is no risk in Asmara. Resistance to chloroquine and sulfadoxine–pyrimethamine reported.

Recommended prevention in risk areas: **IV**

ESTONIA

Yellow fever

Country requirement: no

Yellow fever vaccine recommendation: no

ETHIOPIA

Yellow fever

Country requirement: a yellow fever vaccination certificate is required from travellers over 1 year of age arriving from countries with risk of yellow fever transmission.

Yellow fever vaccine recommendation: yes

Recommended for all travellers aged 9 months or over, except as mentioned below.

Generally not recommended[1] for travellers whose itineraries are limited to the Afar and Somali provinces (Map).

Malaria: Malaria risk – approximately 60% *P. falciparum*, 40% *P. vivax* – exists throughout the year in the whole country below 2000 m. *P. falciparum* resistance to chloroquine and sulfadoxine–pyrimethamine reported. *P. vivax* resistance to chloroquine reported. There is no malaria risk in Addis Ababa.

Recommended prevention in risk areas: **IV**

FALKLAND ISLANDS (MALVINAS)

Yellow fever

Country requirement: no

Yellow fever vaccine recommendation: no

FAROE ISLANDS

Yellow fever

Country requirement: no

Yellow fever vaccine recommendation: no

FIJI

Yellow fever

Country requirement: a yellow fever vaccination certificate is required from travellers over 1 year of age arriving from countries with risk of yellow fever transmission.

Yellow fever vaccine recommendation: no

---

[1] Yellow fever vaccination is *generally not recommended* in areas where there is low potential for exposure to yellow fever virus. However, vaccination might be considered for a small subset of travellers to these areas, who are at increased risk of exposure to yellow fever virus (e.g. prolonged travel, extensive exposure to mosquitoes, inability to avoid mosquito bites). When considering vaccination, any traveller must take into account the risk of being infected with yellow fever virus, country entry requirements, as well as individual risk factors (e.g. age, immune status) for serious vaccine-associated adverse events.

FINLAND

Yellow fever

Country requirement: no

Yellow fever vaccine recommendation: no

FRANCE

Yellow fever

Country requirement: no

Yellow fever vaccine recommendation: no

FRENCH GUIANA

Yellow fever

Country requirement: a yellow fever vaccination certificate is required from all travellers over 1 year of age.

Yellow fever vaccine recommendation: yes

Malaria: Malaria risk – *P. falciparum* (45%), *P. vivax* (55%) – is high throughout the year in nine municipalities of the territory bordering Brazil (Oiapoque river valley) and Suriname (Maroni river valley). In the other 13 municipalities, transmission risk is low or negligible. Multidrug-resistant *P. falciparum* reported in areas influenced by Brazilian migration

Recommended prevention in risk areas: **IV**

FRENCH POLYNESIA

Yellow fever

Country requirement: no.

Yellow fever vaccine recommendation: no

GABON

Yellow fever

Country requirement: a yellow fever vaccination certificate is required from all travellers over 1 year of age.

Yellow fever vaccine recommendation: yes

Malaria: Malaria risk due predominantly to *P. falciparum* exists throughout the year in the whole country. Resistance to chloroquine and sulfadoxine–pyrimethamine reported.

Recommended prevention: **IV**

GALAPAGOS ISLANDS *see* EQUADOR

GAMBIA

Yellow fever

Country requirement: a yellow fever vaccination certificate is required from travellers over 1 year of age arriving from countries with risk of yellow fever transmission.

Yellow fever vaccine recommendation: yes

Malaria: Malaria risk due predominantly to *P. falciparum* exists throughout the year in the whole country. Resistance to chloroquine and sulfadoxine–pyrimethamine reported.

Recommended prevention: **IV**

GEORGIA

Yellow fever

Country requirement: no

Yellow fever vaccine recommendation: no

Malaria: Limited malaria risk due exclusively to *P. vivax* exists focally from June to October inclusive in the eastern part of the country bordering Azerbaijan.

Recommended prevention in risk areas: **I**

GERMANY

Yellow fever

Country requirement: no

Yellow fever vaccine recommendation: no

GHANA

Yellow fever

Country requirement: a yellow fever vaccination certificate is required from all travellers over 9 months of age.

Yellow fever vaccine recommendation: yes

Malaria: Malaria risk due predominantly to *P. falciparum* exists throughout the year in the whole country. Resistance to chloroquine and sulfadoxine–pyrimethamine reported.

Recommended prevention: **IV**

GIBRALTAR

Yellow fever

Country requirement: no

Yellow fever vaccine recommendation: no

GREECE

Yellow fever

Country requirement: no

Yellow fever vaccine recommendation: no

GREENLAND

Yellow fever

Country requirement: no

Yellow fever vaccine recommendation: no

GRENADA

Yellow fever

Country requirement: a yellow fever vaccination certificate is required from travellers over 1 year of age arriving from countries with risk of yellow fever transmission.

Yellow fever vaccine recommendation: no

GUADELOUPE

Yellow fever

Country requirement: a yellow fever vaccination certificate is required from travellers over 1 year of age arriving from countries with risk of yellow fever transmission.

Yellow fever vaccine recommendation: no

GUAM

Yellow fever

Country requirement: no

Yellow fever vaccine recommendation: no

GUATEMALA

Yellow fever

Country requirement: a yellow fever vaccination certificate is required from travellers over 1 year of age arriving from countries with risk of yellow fever transmission.

Yellow fever vaccine recommendation: no

Malaria: Malaria risk due predominantly to *P. vivax* exists throughout the year below 1500 m. There is moderate risk in the departments of Escuintla and Izabal, and low risk in Alta Verapaz, Baja Verapaz, Chiquimala, Petén, Suchitepéquez and Zacapa.

Recommended prevention in risk areas: **II**

GUINEA

Yellow fever

Country requirement: a yellow fever vaccination certificate is required from travellers over 1 year of age arriving from countries with risk of yellow fever transmission.

Yellow fever vaccine recommendation: yes

Malaria: Malaria risk due predominantly to *P. falciparum* exists throughout the year in the whole country. Resistance to chloroquine reported.

Recommended prevention: **IV**

GUINEA-BISSAU

Yellow fever

Country requirement: a yellow fever vaccination certificate is required from all travellers over 1 year of age

Yellow fever vaccine recommendation: yes

Malaria: Malaria risk due predominantly to *P. falciparum* exists throughout the year in the whole country. Resistance to chloroquine and sulfadoxine–pyrimethamine reported.

Recommended prevention: **IV**

GUYANA

Yellow fever

Country requirement: a yellow fever vaccination certificate is required from all travellers over one year of age arriving from countries with risk of yellow fever transmission with the exception of Argentina, Paraguay, Suriname and Trinidad and Tobago.

Yellow fever vaccine recommendation: yes

Malaria: Malaria risk – *P. vivax* (44%), *P. falciparum* (45%), mixed infections (10%) – is high throughout the year in all parts of the interior. Risk is highest in Regions 1, 2, 4, 7, 8, 9 and 10, and very low in Regions 3, 5 and 6. Sporadic cases of malaria have been reported from the densely populated coastal belt. Chloroquine-resistant *P. falciparum* reported.

Recommended prevention in risk areas: **IV**

HAITI

Yellow fever

Country requirement: a yellow fever vaccination certificate is required from travellers arriving from countries with risk of yellow fever transmission.

Yellow fever vaccine recommendation: no

Malaria: Malaria risk due exclusively to *P. falciparum* exists throughout the year in the whole country. No *P. falciparum* resistance to chloroquine reported.

Recommended prevention: **II; or IV if chloroquine is not available pre-travel**

HONDURAS

Yellow fever

Country requirement: a yellow fever vaccination certificate is required from travellers over 1 year of age arriving from countries with risk of yellow fever transmission.

Yellow fever vaccine recommendation: no

Malaria: Malaria risk due to *P. vivax* (85%), *P. falciparum* (14%) and mixed infections (1%). *P. vivax* transmission risk is high in the departments of Gracias a Dios and Islas de la Bahía, and moderate in Atlántida, Colón, Olancho, Valle and Yoro. *P. falciparum* transmission risk is high in Gracias a Dios, and a few cases are also reported in Atlántida, Colon, Islas de la Bahía, Olancho and Yoro.

Recommended prevention in risk areas: **II**

HONG KONG SPECIAL ADMINISTRATIVE REGION OF CHINA see CHINA, HONG KONG SAR

HUNGARY

Yellow fever

Country requirement: no

Yellow fever vaccine recommendation: no

ICELAND

Yellow fever

Country requirement: no

Yellow fever vaccine recommendation: no

INDIA

Yellow fever

Country requirement: anyone (except infants up to the age of 9 months) arriving by air or sea without a yellow fever vaccination certificate is detained in isolation for up to 6 days if that person (i) arrives within 6 days of departure from an area with risk of yellow fever transmission, or (ii) has been in such an area in transit (except those passengers and members of the crew who, while in transit through an airport situated in an area with risk of yellow fever transmission, remained within the airport premises during the period of their entire stay and the Health Officer agrees to such exemption), or (iii) arrives on a ship that started from or touched at any port in an area with risk of yellow fever transmission up to 30 days before its arrival in India, unless such a ship has been disinsected in accordance with the procedure laid down by WHO, or (iv) arrives on an aircraft that has been in an area with risk of yellow fever transmission and has not been disinsected in accordance with the Indian Aircraft Public Health Rules, 1954, or as recommended by WHO.

The following are regarded as countries and areas with risk of yellow fever transmission:

Africa: Angola, Benin, Burkina Faso, Burundi, Cameroon, Central African Republic, Chad, Congo, Côte d'Ivoire, Democratic Republic of the Congo, Equatorial Guinea, Ethiopia, Gabon, Gambia, Ghana, Guinea, Guinea-Bissau, Kenya, Liberia, Mali, Niger, Nigeria, Rwanda, Senegal, Sierra Leone, Sudan, Togo, Uganda, Zambia.

America: Bolivarian Republic of Venezuela, Brazil, Colombia, Ecuador, French Guiana, Guyana, Panama, Peru, Plurinational State of Bolivia, Suriname and Trinidad and Tobago.

Note. When a case of yellow fever is reported from any country, that country is regarded by the Government of India as a country with risk of yellow fever transmission and is added to the above list.

Yellow fever vaccine recommendations: no

Malaria: Malaria risk exists throughout the year in the whole country at altitudes below 2000 m, with overall 40–50% of cases due to *P. falciparum* and the remainder due to *P. vivax*. There is no transmission in parts of the states of Himachal Pradesh, Jammu and Kashmir, and Sikkim. Risk of falciparum malaria and drug resistance are relatively higher in the north-eastern states, in the Andaman and Nicobar Islands, Chhattisgarh, Gujarat, Jharkhand, Karnataka (with the exception of the city of Bangalore) Madhya Pradesh, Maharasthra (with the exception of the cities of Mumbai, Nagpur, Nasik and Pune), Orissa and

West Bengal (with the exception of the city of Kolkata). *P. falciparum* resistance to chloroquine and sulfadoxine–pyrimethamine reported.

Recommended prevention in risk areas: **III**; in the listed higher risk areas: **IV**

INDONESIA

Yellow fever

Country requirement: a yellow fever vaccination certificate is required from travellers over 9 months of age arriving from countries with risk of yellow fever transmission.

Yellow fever vaccine recommendation: no

Malaria: Malaria risk exists throughout the year in all areas of the five eastern provinces of East Nusa Tenggara, Maluku, North Maluku, Papua and West Papua. In other parts of the country, there is malaria risk in some districts, except in Jakarta Municipality, in big cities, and within the areas of the main tourist resorts. *P. falciparum* resistant to chloroquine and sulfadoxine–pyrimethamine reported. *P. vivax* resistant to chloroquine reported. Human *P. knowlesi* infection reported in the province of Kalimantan.

Recommended prevention in risk areas: **IV**

IRAN (ISLAMIC REPUBLIC OF)

Yellow fever

Country requirement: a yellow fever vaccination certificate is required from travellers arriving from countries with risk of yellow fever transmission.

Yellow fever vaccine recommendation: no

Malaria: Malaria risk due to *P. vivax* and *P. falciparum* exists from March to November inclusive in rural areas of the provinces of Hormozgan and Kerman (tropical part) and the southern part of Sistan-Baluchestan. *P. falciparum* resistant to chloroquine and sulfadoxine–pyrimethamine reported.

Recommended prevention in risk areas: **IV**

IRAQ

Yellow fever

Country requirement: a yellow fever vaccination certificate is required from travellers arriving from countries with risk of yellow fever transmission.

Yellow fever vaccine recommendation: no

Malaria: Limited malaria risk due exclusively to *P. vivax* – may exist from May to November inclusive in areas in the north below 1500 m (Duhok, Erbil and Sulaimaniya provinces). No indigenous cases reported since 2009.

Recommended prevention in risk areas: **I**

IRELAND

Yellow fever

Country requirement: no

Yellow fever vaccine recommendation: no

ISRAEL

Yellow fever

Country requirement: no

Yellow fever vaccine recommendation: no

ITALY

Yellow fever

Country requirement: no

Yellow fever vaccine recommendation: no

JAMAICA

Yellow fever

Country requirement: a yellow fever vaccination certificate is required from travellers over 1 year of age arriving from countries with risk of yellow fever transmission.

Yellow fever vaccine recommendation: no

Malaria: Very limited risk of *P. falciparum* malaria may occur in the Kingston St Andrew Parish.

Recommended prevention in risk areas: **I**

JAPAN

Yellow fever

Country requirement: no

Yellow fever vaccine recommendation: no

JORDAN

Yellow fever

Country requirement: a yellow fever vaccination certificate is required from travellers over 1 year of age arriving from countries with risk of yellow fever transmission.

Yellow fever vaccine recommendation: no

KAZAKHSTAN

Yellow fever

Country requirement: a yellow fever vaccination certificate is required from travellers arriving from countries with risk of yellow fever transmission.

Yellow fever vaccine recommendation: no

KENYA

Yellow fever

Country requirement: a yellow fever vaccination certificate is required from travellers over 1 year of age arriving from countries with risk of yellow fever transmission.

Yellow fever vaccine recommendation: yes

Recommended for all travellers aged 9 months or over, except as mentioned below.

Generally not recommended[1] for travellers whose itineraries are limited to the following areas: the entire North Eastern Province; the states of Kilifi, Kwale, Lamu, Malindi and Tanariver in the Coastal Province; and the cities of Nairobi and Mombasa (Map).

Malaria: Malaria risk due predominantly to *P. falciparum* exists throughout the year in the whole country. Normally, there is little risk in the city of Nairobi and in the highlands (above 2500 m) of Central, Eastern, Nyanza, Rift Valley and Western provinces. Resistance to chloroquine and sulfadoxine–pyrimethamine reported.

Recommended prevention: **IV**

KIRIBATI

Yellow fever

Country requirement: a yellow fever vaccination certificate is required from travellers over 1 year of age arriving from countries with risk of yellow fever transmission.

Yellow fever vaccine recommendation: no

---

[1] Yellow fever vaccination is *generally not recommended* in areas where there is low potential for exposure to yellow fever virus. However, vaccination might be considered for a small subset of travellers to these areas, who are at increased risk of exposure to yellow fever virus (e.g. prolonged travel, extensive exposure to mosquitoes, inability to avoid mosquito bites). When considering vaccination, any traveller must take into account the risk of being infected with yellow fever virus, country entry requirements, as well as individual risk factors (e.g. age, immune status) for serious vaccine-associated adverse events.

KOREA, REPUBLIC OF, *see* REPUBLIC OF KOREA

KOREA, DEMOCRATIC PEOPLE'S REPUBLIC OF, *see* DEMOCRATIC PEOPLE'S REPUBLIC OF KOREA

KUWAIT

Yellow fever

Country requirement: no

Yellow fever vaccine recommendation: no

KYRGYZSTAN

Yellow fever

Country requirement: no

Yellow fever vaccine recommendation: no

Malaria: Malaria risk due exclusively to *P. vivax* exists from June to October inclusive in some southern and western parts of the country, mainly in areas bordering Tajikistan and Uzbekistan (Batken, Jalal-Abad and Osh regions) and in the outskirts of Bishkek.

Recommended prevention in risk areas: **I**

LAO PEOPLE'S DEMOCRATIC REPUBLIC

Yellow fever

Country requirement: a yellow fever vaccination certificate is required from travellers arriving from countries with risk of yellow fever transmission.

Yellow fever vaccine recommendation: no

Malaria: Malaria risk due predominantly to *P. falciparum* exists throughout the year in the whole country except in Vientiane. *P. falciparum* resistant to chloroquine and sulfadoxine–pyrimethamine reported.

Recommended prevention in risk areas: **IV**

LATVIA

Yellow fever

Country requirement: no

Yellow fever vaccine recommendation: no

LEBANON

Yellow fever

Country requirement: a yellow fever vaccination certificate is required from travellers over 6 months

of age arriving from countries with risk of yellow fever transmission.

Yellow fever vaccine recommendation: no

LESOTHO

Yellow fever

Country requirement: a yellow fever vaccination certificate is required from travellers over 9 months of age arriving from countries with risk of yellow fever transmission.

Yellow fever vaccine recommendation: no

LIBERIA

Yellow fever

Country requirement: a yellow fever vaccination certificate is required from all travellers over 1 year of age.

Yellow fever vaccine recommendation: yes

Malaria: Malaria risk due predominantly to *P. falciparum* exists throughout the year in the whole country. Resistance to chloroquine and sulfadoxine–pyrimethamine reported.

Recommended prevention: **IV**

LIBYAN ARAB JAMAHIRIYA

Yellow fever

Country requirement: a yellow fever vaccination certificate is required from travellers arriving from countries with risk of yellow fever transmission.

Yellow fever vaccine recommendation: no

LIECHTENSTEIN

Yellow fever

Country requirement: no

Yellow fever vaccine recommendation: no

LITHUANIA

Yellow fever

Country requirement: no

Yellow fever vaccine recommendation: no

LUXEMBOURG

Yellow fever

Country requirement: no

Yellow fever vaccine recommendation: no

MACAO SPECIAL ADMINISTRATIVE REGION OF CHINA *see* CHINA, MACAO SAR

MADAGASCAR

Yellow fever

Country requirement: a yellow fever vaccination certificate is required from travellers arriving from countries with risk of yellow fever transmission.

Yellow fever vaccine recommendation: no

Malaria: Malaria risk due predominantly to *P. falciparum* exists throughout the year in the whole country, with the highest risk in coastal areas. Resistance to chloroquine reported.

Recommended prevention: **IV**

MADEIRA ISLANDS *see* PORTUGAL

MALAWI

Yellow fever

Country requirement: a yellow fever vaccination certificate is required from travellers over 1 year of age arriving from countries with risk of yellow fever transmission.

Yellow fever vaccine recommendation: no

Malaria: Malaria risk due predominantly to *P. falciparum* exists throughout the year in the whole country. Resistance to chloroquine and sulfadoxine–pyrimethamine reported.

Recommended prevention: **IV**

MALAYSIA

Yellow fever

Country requirement: a yellow fever vaccination certificate is required from travellers over 1 year of age arriving from countries with risk of yellow fever transmission.

Yellow fever vaccine recommendation: no

Malaria: Malaria risk exists only in limited foci in the deep hinterland. Urban and coastal areas are free from malaria. *P. falciparum* resistant to chloroquine and sulfadoxine–pyrimethamine reported. Human *P. knowlesi* infection reported. *P. vivax* resistance to chloroquine reported.

Recommended prevention in risk areas: **IV**

MALDIVES

Yellow fever

Country requirement: a yellow fever vaccination certificate is required from travellers over 1 year of age arriving from countries with risk of yellow fever transmission.

Yellow fever vaccine recommendation: no

MALI

Yellow fever

Country requirement: a yellow fever vaccination certificate is required from all travellers over 1 year of age.

Yellow fever vaccine recommendation: yes

Recommended for all travellers aged 9 months or over going to areas south of the Sahara Desert (Map).

Not recommended for travellers whose itineraries are limited to areas in the Sahara Desert (Map).

Malaria: Malaria risk due predominantly to *P. falciparum* exists throughout the year in the whole country. Resistance to chloroquine and sulfadoxine–pyrimethamine reported.

Recommended prevention: **IV**

MALTA

Yellow fever

Country requirement: a yellow fever vaccination certificate is required from travellers over 9 months of age arriving from countries with risk of yellow fever transmission. If indicated on epidemiological grounds, infants under 9 months of age are subject to isolation or surveillance if coming from an area with risk of yellow fever transmission.

Yellow fever vaccine recommendation: no

MARSHALL ISLANDS

Yellow fever

Country requirement: no

Yellow fever vaccine recommendation: no

MARTINIQUE

Yellow fever

Country requirement: a yellow fever vaccination certificate is required from travellers over 1 year of age arriving from countries with risk of yellow fever transmission.

Yellow fever vaccine recommendation: no

MAURITANIA

Yellow fever

Country requirement: a yellow fever vaccination certificate is required from travellers over 1 year of age arriving from countries with risk of yellow fever transmission.

Yellow fever vaccine recommendation: yes:

Recommended for all travellers aged 9 months or over travelling to areas south of the Sahara Desert (Map).

Not recommended for travellers whose itineraries are limited to areas in the Sahara Desert (Map).

Malaria: Malaria risk due predominantly to *P. falciparum* exists throughout the year in the whole country, except in northern areas (Dakhlet-Nouadhibou and Tiris-Zemour). In Adrar and Inchiri there is malaria risk during the rainy season (from July to October inclusive). Resistance to chloroquine reported.

Recommended prevention in risk areas: **IV**

MAURITIUS

Yellow fever

Country requirement: a yellow fever vaccination certificate is required from travellers over 1 year of age arriving from countries with risk of yellow fever transmission.

Yellow fever vaccine recommendation: no

MAYOTTE (FRENCH TERRITORIAL COLLECTIVITY)

Yellow fever

Country requirement: no

Yellow fever vaccine recommendation: no

Malaria: Malaria risk due predominantly to *P. falciparum* exists throughout the year. Resistance to chloroquine and sulfadoxine–pyrimethamine reported.

Recommended prevention: **IV**

MEXICO

Yellow fever

Country requirement: no

Yellow fever vaccine recommendation: no

Malaria: Malaria risk due almost exclusively to *P. vivax* exists throughout the year in some rural areas that are not often visited by tourists. There is moderate risk in some localities in the states of Chiapas and Oaxaca; very low-risk localities are also found in the states of Chihuahua, Durango, Nayarit, Quintana Roo and Sinaloa.

Recommended prevention in risk areas: **II**

MICRONESIA (FEDERATED STATES OF)

Yellow fever

Country requirement: no

Yellow fever vaccine recommendation: no

MONACO

Yellow fever

Country requirement: no

Yellow fever vaccine recommendation: no

MONGOLIA

Yellow fever

Country requirement: no

Yellow fever vaccine recommendation: no

MONTENEGRO

Yellow fever

Country requirement: no

Yellow fever vaccine recommendation: no

MONTSERRAT

Yellow fever

Country requirement: a yellow fever vaccination certificate is required from travellers over 1 year of age arriving from countries with risk of yellow fever transmission.

Yellow fever vaccine recommendation: no

MOROCCO

Yellow fever

Country requirement: no

Yellow fever vaccine recommendation: no

MOZAMBIQUE

Yellow fever

Country requirement: a yellow fever vaccination certificate is required from travellers over 1 year of age arriving from countries with risk of yellow fever transmission.

Yellow fever vaccine recommendation: no

Malaria: Malaria risk due predominantly to *P. falciparum* exists throughout the year in the whole country. Resistance to chloroquine and sulfadoxine–pyrimethamine reported.

Recommended prevention: **IV**

MYANMAR (FORMERLY BURMA)

Yellow fever

Country requirement: a yellow fever vaccination certificate is required from travellers arriving from countries with risk of yellow fever transmission. Nationals and residents of Myanmar are required to possess certificates of vaccination on their departure to an area with risk of yellow fever transmission.

Yellow fever vaccine recommendation: no

Malaria: Malaria risk due predominantly to *P. falciparum* exists throughout the year at altitudes below 1000 m, excluding the main urban areas of Mandalay and Yangon. Risk is highest in remote rural, hilly and forested areas. *P. falciparum* resistant to chloroquine and sulfadoxine–pyrimethamine reported. Mefloquine resistance reported in Kayin state and the eastern part of Shan state. *P. vivax* resistance to chloroquine reported. Human *P. knowlesi* infection reported.

Recommended prevention in risk areas: **IV**

NAMIBIA

Yellow fever

Country requirement: a yellow fever vaccination certificate is required from travellers arriving from countries with risk of yellow fever transmission. The countries, or parts of countries, included in the endemic zones in Africa and South America are regarded as areas with risk of yellow fever transmission. Travellers who are on scheduled flights that originated outside the countries with risk of yellow fever transmission, but who have been in transit through these areas, are not required to possess a certificate provided that they remained at the scheduled airport or in the adjacent town during transit. All travellers whose flights originated in countries with risk of yellow fever transmission or who have been in transit through these countries on unscheduled flights are required to possess a certificate. The certificate is not insisted upon in the case of children under 1 year of age, but such infants may be subject to surveillance.

Yellow fever vaccine recommendation: no

Malaria: Malaria risk due predominantly to P. *falciparum* exists from November to June inclusive in the following regions: Ohangwena, Omaheke, Omusati, Oshana, Oshikoto and Otjozondjupa. Risk exists throughout the year along the Kunene river and in Caprivi and Kavango regions. Resistance to chloroquine and sulfadoxine–pyrimethamine reported.

Recommended prevention in risk areas: **IV**

NAURU

Yellow fever

Country requirement: a yellow fever vaccination certificate is required from travellers over 1 year of age arriving from countries with risk of yellow fever transmission.

Yellow fever vaccine recommendation: no

NEPAL

Yellow fever

Country requirement: a yellow fever vaccination certificate is required from travellers arriving from countries with risk of yellow fever transmission.

Yellow fever vaccine recommendation: no

Malaria: Malaria risk due predominantly to P. *vivax* exists throughout the year in rural areas of the 20 Terai districts bordering India, with occasional outbreaks of P. *falciparum* from July to October inclusive. Seasonal transmission of P. *vivax* takes place in 45 districts of the inner Terai and mid-hills. P. *falciparum* resistant to chloroquine and sulfadoxine–pyrimethamine reported.

Recommended prevention in risk areas: **III**

NETHERLANDS

Yellow fever

Country requirement: no

Yellow fever vaccine recommendation: no

NETHERLANDS ANTILLES (BONAIRE, CURAÇAO, SABA, ST EUSTASIUS, ST MARTIN)

Yellow fever

Country requirement: a yellow fever vaccination certificate is required from travellers over 6 months of age arriving from countries with risk of yellow fever transmission.

Yellow fever vaccine recommendation: no

NEW CALEDONIA AND DEPENDENCIES

Yellow fever

Country requirement: a yellow fever vaccination certificate is required from travellers over 1 year of age arriving from countries with risk of yellow fever transmission.

Note. In the event of an epidemic threat to the territory, a specific vaccination certificate may be required.

Yellow fever vaccine recommendation: no

NEW ZEALAND

Yellow fever

Country requirement: no

Yellow fever vaccine recommendation: no

NICARAGUA

Yellow fever

Country requirement: a yellow fever vaccination certificate is required from travellers over 1 year of age arriving from countries with risk of yellow fever transmission.

Yellow fever vaccine recommendation: no

Malaria: Low malaria risk due predominantly to P. *vivax* (85%) exists throughout the year in a number of municipalities in Chinandega, Léon, Managua, Matagalpa, Región Autónoma del Atlántico Norte and Región Autónoma del Atlántico Sur. Cases are reported from other municipalities in the central and western departments but the risk in these areas is considered to be very low or negligible. No chloroquine-resistant P. *falciparum* reported.

Recommended prevention in risk areas: **II**

NIGER

Yellow fever

Country requirement: a yellow fever vaccination certificate is required from all travellers over 1 year of age and recommended for travellers departing Niger.

Yellow fever vaccine recommendation: yes:

Recommended for all travellers aged 9 months or over travelling to areas south of the Sahara Desert (Map).

Not recommended for travellers whose itineraries are limited to areas in the Sahara Desert (Map).

Malaria: Malaria risk due predominantly to *P. falciparum* exists throughout the year in the whole country. Chloroquine-resistant *P. falciparum* reported.

Recommended prevention: **IV**

NIGERIA

Yellow fever

Country requirement: a yellow fever vaccination certificate is required from travellers over 1 year of age arriving from countries with risk of yellow fever transmission.

Yellow fever vaccine recommendation: yes

Malaria: Malaria risk due predominantly to *P. falciparum* exists throughout the year in the whole country. Resistance to chloroquine and sulfadoxine–pyrimethamine reported.

Recommended prevention: **IV**

NIUE

Yellow fever

Country requirement: a yellow fever vaccination certificate is required from travellers over 9 months of age arriving from countries with risk of yellow fever transmission.

Yellow fever vaccine recommendation: no

NORFOLK ISLAND *see* AUSTRALIA

NORTHERN MARIANA ISLANDS

Yellow fever

Country requirement: no

Yellow fever vaccine recommendation: no

NORWAY

Yellow fever

Country requirement: no

Yellow fever vaccine recommendation: no

OMAN

Yellow fever

Country requirement: a yellow fever vaccination certificate is required from travellers over 1 year of age arriving from countries with risk of yellow fever transmission.

Yellow fever vaccine recommendation: no

Malaria: Sporadic transmission of *P. falciparum* and *P. vivax* may occur subsequent to international importations of parasites. In 2010, local outbreaks of *P. falciparum* and *P. vivax* were reported in North Sharqiya region.

Recommended prevention: **I** (mosquito bite prevention only)

PAKISTAN

Yellow fever

Country requirement: a yellow fever vaccination certificate is required from travellers arriving from any part of a country in which there is a risk of yellow fever transmission; infants under 6 months of age are exempt if the mother's vaccination certificate shows that she was vaccinated before the birth of the child.

Yellow fever vaccine recommendation: no

Malaria: Malaria risk – *P. vivax* and *P. falciparum* – exists throughout the year in the whole country below 2000 m. *P. falciparum* resistant to chloroquine and sulfadoxine–pyrimethamine reported.

Recommended prevention in risk areas: **IV**

PALAU

Yellow fever

Country requirement: no

Yellow fever vaccine recommendation: no

PANAMA

Yellow fever

Country requirement: a yellow fever vaccination certificate is required from all travellers arriving from countries with risk of yellow fever transmission.

Yellow fever vaccination recommendation: yes:

Recommended for all travellers aged 9 months or over travelling to all mainland areas east of the Canal Zone, (the entire comarcas of Emberá and Kuna Yala, the province of Darién and areas of the provinces of Colón and Panama that are east of the Canal Zone) (Map).

Not recommended[1] for travellers whose itineraries are limited to areas west of the canal zone, the city

---

[1] Yellow fever vaccination is *generally not recommended* in areas where there is low potential for exposure to yellow fever virus. However, vaccination might be considered for a small subset of travellers to these areas, who are at increased risk of exposure to yellow fever virus (e.g. prolonged travel, extensive exposure to mosquitoes, inability to avoid mosquito bites). When considering vaccination, any traveller must take into account the risk of being infected with yellow fever virus, country entry requirements, as well as individual risk factors (e.g. age, immune status) for serious vaccine-associated adverse events.

of Panama, the canal zone itself, and the Balboa and San Blas Islands (Map).

Malaria: Malaria risk due predominantly to *P. vivax* (99%) exists throughout the year in provinces and comarcas along the Atlantic coast and the borders with Costa Rica and Colombia: Bocas del Toro, Chiriquí, Colón, Darién, Kuna Yala, Ngäbe Buglé, Panama and Veraguas. In Panama City, in the Canal Zone, and in the other provinces there is no or negligible risk of transmission. Chloroquine-resistant *P. falciparum* has been reported in Darién and San Blas.

Recommended prevention in risk areas: **II**; in eastern endemic areas: **IV**

PAPUA NEW GUINEA

Yellow fever

Country requirement: a yellow fever vaccination certificate is required from travellers over 1 year of age arriving from countries with risk of yellow fever transmission.

Yellow fever vaccine recommendation: no

Malaria: Malaria risk due predominantly to *P. falciparum* exists throughout the year in the whole country below 1800 m. *P. falciparum* resistant to chloroquine and sulfadoxine–pyrimethamine reported. *P. vivax* resistant to chloroquine reported.

Recommended prevention in risk areas: **IV**

PARAGUAY

Yellow fever

Country requirement: a yellow fever vaccination certificate is required from travellers over 1 year of age arriving from countries with risk of yellow fever transmission.

Yellow fever vaccine recommendation: yes

Recommended for all travellers aged 9 months or over, except as mentioned below.

Generally not recommended[1] for travellers whose itineraries are limited to the city of Asunción.

Malaria: Malaria risk due almost exclusively to *P. vivax* is moderate in certain municipalities of the departments of Alto Paraná and Caaguazú. In other departments there is no or negligible transmission risk.

Recommended prevention in risk areas: **II**

PERU

Yellow fever

Country requirement: no

Yellow fever vaccine recommendation: yes

Recommended for all travellers aged 9 months or over going to the following areas at altitudes below 2300 m: the entire regions of Amazonas, Loreto, Madre de Dios, San Martin and Ucayali, and designated areas (Map) of the following regions: far-north-eastern Ancash; northern Apurímac; northern and north-eastern Ayacucho; northern and eastern Cajamarca; north-western, northern, and north-eastern Cusco; far-northern Huancavelica; northern, central and eastern Huánuco; northern and eastern Junín; eastern La Libertad; central and eastern Pasco; eastern Piura; and northern Puno.

Generally not recommended[1] for travellers whose itineraries are limited to the following areas west of the Andes: the entire regions of Lambayeque and Tumbes and the designated areas (Map) of western Piura and west-central Cajamarca.

Not recommended for travellers whose itineraries are limited to the following areas: all areas above 2300 m altitude, areas west of the Andes not listed above, the cities of Cuzco and Lima, Machu Picchu, and the Inca Trail (Map).

Malaria: Malaria risk – *P. vivax* (89%), *P. falciparum* (11%) – exists throughout the year in rural areas at altitudes below 2000 m. The 23 highest-risk districts are concentrated in the regions of Ayacucho, Junín, Loreto, Madre de Dios, Piura, San Martin and Tumbes. Ninety-nine percent of *P. falciparum* cases are reported from Loreto, which is situated in the Amazon and contains 18 of the highest-risk districts in the country. *P. falciparum* resistance to chloroquine and sulfadoxine–pyrimethamine reported. *P. vivax* resistance to chloroquine reported.

Recommended prevention in risk areas: **II** in *P. vivax* risk areas; **IV** in Loreto

[1] Yellow fever vaccination is *generally not recommended* in areas where there is low potential for exposure to yellow fever virus. However, vaccination might be considered for a small subset of travellers to these areas, who are at increased risk of exposure to yellow fever virus (e.g. prolonged travel, extensive exposure to mosquitoes, inability to avoid mosquito bites). When considering vaccination, any traveller must take into account the risk of being infected with yellow fever virus, country entry requirements, as well as individual risk factors (e.g. age, immune status) for serious vaccine-associated adverse events.

PHILIPPINES

Yellow fever

Country requirement: a yellow fever vaccination certificate is required from travellers over 1 year of age arriving from countries with risk of yellow fever transmission.

Yellow fever vaccine recommendation: no

Malaria: Malaria risk exists throughout the year in areas below 600 m, except in the 22 provinces of Aklan, Albay, Benguet, Biliran, Bohol, Camiguin, Capiz, Catanduanes, Cavite, Cebu, Guimaras, Iloilo, Northern Leyte, Southern Leyte, Marinduque, Masbate, Eastern Samar, Northern Samar, Western Samar, Siquijor, Sorsogon, Surigao Del Norte and metropolitan Manila. No risk is considered to exist in urban areas or in the plains. *P. falciparum* resistant to chloroquine and sulfadoxine–pyrimethamine reported. Human *P. knowlesi* infection reported in the province of Palawan.

Recommended prevention in risk areas: **IV**

PITCAIRN

Yellow fever

Country requirement: a yellow fever vaccination certificate is required from travellers over 1 year of age arriving from countries with risk of yellow fever transmission.

Yellow fever vaccine recommendation: no

POLAND

Yellow fever

Country requirement: no

Yellow fever vaccine recommendation: no

PORTUGAL

Yellow fever

Country requirement: no

Yellow fever vaccine recommendation: no

PUERTO RICO

Yellow fever

Country requirement: no

Yellow fever vaccine recommendation: no

QATAR

Yellow fever

Country requirement: no

Yellow fever vaccine recommendation: no

REPUBLIC OF KOREA

Yellow fever

Country requirement: no

Yellow fever vaccine recommendation: no

Malaria: Limited malaria risk due exclusively to *P. vivax* exists mainly in the northern areas of Gangwon-do and Gyeonggi-do Provinces and Incheon City (towards the Demilitarized Zone or DMZ).

Recommended prevention in risk areas: **I**

REPUBLIC OF MOLDOVA

Yellow fever

Country requirement: no

Yellow fever vaccine recommendation: no

REUNION

Yellow fever

Country requirement: a yellow fever vaccination certificate is required from travellers over 1 year of age arriving from countries with risk of yellow fever transmission.

Yellow fever vaccine recommendation: no

ROMANIA

Yellow fever

Country requirement: no

Yellow fever vaccine recommendation: no

RUSSIAN FEDERATION

Yellow fever

Country requirement: a yellow fever vaccination certificate is required from travellers over 9 months of age arriving from countries with risk of yellow fever transmission.

Yellow fever vaccine recommendation: no

Malaria: Very limited malaria risk due exclusively to *P. vivax* may exist in areas under influence of intense migration from southern countries in the Commonwealth of Independent States.

Recommended prevention: **none**

RWANDA

Yellow fever

Country requirement: a yellow fever vaccination certificate is required from all travellers over 1 year of age.

Yellow fever vaccine recommendation: yes

Malaria: Malaria risk due predominantly to *P. falciparum* exists throughout the year in the whole country. Resistance to chloroquine and sulfadoxine–pyrimethamine reported.

Recommended prevention: **IV**

SAINT HELENA

Yellow fever

Country requirement: a yellow fever vaccination certificate is required from travellers over 1 year of age arriving from countries with risk of yellow fever transmission.

Yellow fever vaccine recommendation: no

SAINT KITTS AND NEVIS

Yellow fever

Country requirement: a yellow fever vaccination certificate is required from travellers over 1 year of age arriving from countries with risk of yellow fever transmission.

Yellow fever vaccine recommendation: no

SAINT LUCIA

Yellow fever

Country requirement: a yellow fever vaccination certificate is required from travellers over 1 year of age arriving from countries with risk of yellow fever transmission.

Yellow fever vaccine recommendation: no

SAINT PIERRE AND MIQUELON

Yellow fever

Country requirement: no

Yellow fever vaccine recommendation: no

SAINT VINCENT AND THE GRENADINES

Yellow fever

Country requirement: a yellow fever vaccination certificate is required from travellers over 1 year of age arriving from countries with risk of yellow fever transmission.

Yellow fever vaccine recommendation: no

SAMOA

Yellow fever

Country requirement: a yellow fever vaccination certificate is required from travellers over 1 year

of age arriving from countries with risk of yellow fever transmission.

Yellow fever vaccine recommendation: no

SAN MARINO

Yellow fever

Country requirement: no

Yellow fever vaccine recommendation: no

SAO TOME AND PRINCIPE

Yellow fever

Country requirement: a yellow fever vaccination certificate is required from all travellers over 1 year of age.

Yellow fever vaccine recommendation: no

Generally not recommended[1] for travellers to Sao Tome and Principe.

Malaria: Malaria risk due predominantly to *P. falciparum* exists throughout the year. Chloroquine-resistant *P. falciparum* reported

Recommended prevention: **IV**

SAUDI ARABIA

Yellow fever

Country requirement: a yellow fever vaccination certificate is required from all travellers arriving from countries with risk of yellow fever transmission.

Yellow fever vaccine recommendation: no

Malaria: Limited malaria risk due predominantly to *P. falciparum* exists mainly from September to January inclusive in foci along the southern border with Yemen (except in the high altitude areas of Asir Province). No risk in Mecca or Medina cities. Chloroquine-resistant *P. falciparum* reported.

Recommended prevention in risk areas: **IV**

SENEGAL

Yellow fever

Country requirement: a yellow fever vaccination certificate is required from travellers over 9 months

---

[1] Yellow fever vaccination is *generally not recommended* in areas where there is low potential for exposure to yellow fever virus. However, vaccination might be considered for a small subset of travellers to these areas, who are at increased risk of exposure to yellow fever virus (e.g. prolonged travel, extensive exposure to mosquitoes, inability to avoid mosquito bites). When considering vaccination, any traveller must take into account the risk of being infected with yellow fever virus, country entry requirements, as well as individual risk factors (e.g. age, immune status) for serious vaccine-associated adverse events.

of age arriving from countries with risk of yellow fever transmission.

Yellow fever vaccine recommendation: yes

Malaria: Malaria risk due predominantly to *P. falciparum* exists throughout the year in the whole country. There is less risk from January to June inclusive in the central western regions. Resistance to chloroquine and sulfadoxine–pyrimethamine reported.

Recommended prevention: **IV**

SERBIA

Yellow fever

Country requirement: no

Yellow fever vaccine recommendation: no

SEYCHELLES

Yellow fever

Country requirement: a yellow fever vaccination certificate is required from travellers over 1 year of age arriving from countries with risk of yellow fever transmission.

Yellow fever vaccine recommendation: no

SIERRA LEONE

Yellow fever

Country requirement: a yellow fever vaccination certificate is required from all travellers.

Yellow fever vaccine recommendation: yes

Malaria: Malaria risk due predominantly to *P. falciparum* exists throughout the year in the whole country. Resistance to chloroquine and sulfadoxine–pyrimethamine reported.

Recommended prevention: **IV**

SINGAPORE

Yellow fever

Country requirement: certificates of vaccination are required from travellers over 1 year of age who, within the preceding 6 days, have been in or passed through any country with risk of yellow fever transmission.

Yellow fever vaccine recommendation: no

Malaria: One case of human *P. knowlesi* infection reported. Recommended prevention in *P. knowlesi* risk areas: **I**

SLOVAKIA

Yellow fever

Country requirement: no

Yellow fever vaccine recommendation: no

SLOVENIA

Yellow fever

Country requirement: no

Yellow fever vaccine recommendation: no

SOLOMON ISLANDS

Yellow fever

Country requirement: a yellow fever vaccination certificate is required from travellers arriving from countries with risk of yellow fever transmission.

Yellow fever vaccine recommendation: no

Malaria: Malaria risk due predominantly to *P. falciparum* exists throughout the year except in a few outlying eastern and southern islets. *P. falciparum* resistant to chloroquine and sulfadoxine–pyrimethamine reported. *P. vivax* resistance to chloroquine reported.

Recommended prevention in risk areas: **IV**

SOMALIA

Yellow fever

Country requirement: a yellow fever vaccination certificate is required from travellers arriving from countries with risk of yellow fever transmission.

Yellow fever vaccine recommendation: in general, no:

Generally not recommended[1] for travellers going to the following regions: Bakool, Banaadir, Bay, Gado, Galgadud, Hiran, Lower Juba, Middle Juba, Lower Shabelle and Middle Shabelle (Map).

Not recommended for all other areas not listed above.

Malaria: Malaria risk due predominantly to *P. falciparum* exists throughout the year in the whole country. Risk is relatively low and seasonal in the north. It is higher in the central and southern

---

[1] Yellow fever vaccination is *generally not recommended* in areas where there is low potential for exposure to yellow fever virus. However, vaccination might be considered for a small subset of travellers to these areas, who are at increased risk of exposure to yellow fever virus (e.g. prolonged travel, extensive exposure to mosquitoes, inability to avoid mosquito bites). When considering vaccination, any traveller must take into account the risk of being infected with yellow fever virus, country entry requirements, as well as individual risk factors (e.g. age, immune status) for serious vaccine-associated adverse events.

parts of the country. Resistance to chloroquine and sulfadoxine–pyrimethamine reported.

Recommended prevention: **IV**

SOUTH AFRICA

Yellow fever

Country requirement: a yellow fever vaccination certificate is required from travellers over 1 year of age arriving from countries with risk of yellow fever transmission.

Yellow fever vaccine recommendation: no

Malaria: Malaria risk due predominantly to *P. falciparum* exists throughout the year in the low-altitude areas of Mpumalanga Province (including the Kruger National Park), Northern Province and north-eastern KwaZulu-Natal as far south as the Tugela River. Risk is highest from October to May inclusive. Resistance to chloroquine and sulfadoxine–pyrimethamine reported.

Recommended prevention in risk areas: **IV**

SPAIN

Yellow fever

Country requirement: no

Yellow fever vaccine recommendation: no

SRI LANKA

Yellow fever

Country requirement: a yellow fever vaccination certificate is required from travellers over 1 year of age arriving from countries with risk of yellow fever transmission.

Yellow fever vaccine recommendation: no

Malaria: Limited malaria risk – *P. vivax* (88%), *P. falciparum* (12%) – exists throughout the year, except in the districts of Colombo, Galle, Gampaha, Kalutara, Matara and Nuwara Eliya. *P. falciparum* resistant to chloroquine and sulfadoxine–pyrimethamine reported.

Recommended prevention in risk areas: **III**

SUDAN

Yellow fever

Country requirement: a yellow fever vaccination certificate is required from travellers over 9 months of age arriving from countries with risk of yellow fever transmission. A certificate may be required from travellers departing Sudan.

Yellow fever vaccine recommendation: yes

Recommended for all travellers aged 9 months or over travelling to areas south of the Sahara desert (Map).

Not recommended for travellers whose itineraries are limited to areas in the Sahara desert and the city of Khartoum (Map).

Malaria: Malaria risk due predominantly to *P. falciparum* exists throughout the year in the whole country. Risk is low and seasonal in the north. It is higher in the central and southern parts of the country. Malaria risk on the Red Sea coast is very limited. Resistance to chloroquine and sulfadoxine–pyrimethamine reported.

Recommended prevention: **IV**

SURINAME

Yellow fever

Country requirement: a yellow fever vaccination certificate is required from travellers over 1 year of age arriving from countries with risk of yellow fever transmission.

Yellow fever vaccine recommendation: yes

Malaria: Malaria risk – *P. falciparum* (40%), *P. vivax* (58%), mixed infections 2% – continues to decrease in recent years. It occurs throughout the year in the interior of the country beyond the coastal savannah area, with highest risk mainly along the eastern border and in gold-mining areas. In Paramaribo city and the other seven coastal districts, transmission risk is low or negligible. *P. falciparum* resistant to chloroquine, sulfadoxine–pyrimethamine and mefloquine reported. Some decline in quinine sensitivity also reported.

Recommended prevention in risk areas: **IV**

SWAZILAND

Yellow fever

Country requirement: a yellow fever vaccination certificate is required from travellers arriving from countries with risk of yellow fever transmission.

Yellow fever vaccine recommendation: no

Malaria: Malaria risk due predominantly to *P. falciparum* exists throughout the year in all low veld areas (mainly Big Bend, Mhlume, Simunye and Tshaneni). Chloroquine-resistant *P. falciparum* reported.

Recommended prevention in risk areas: **IV**

227

SWEDEN
Yellow fever
Country requirement: no
Yellow fever vaccine recommendation: no

SWITZERLAND
Yellow fever
Country requirement: no
Yellow fever vaccine recommendation: no

SYRIAN ARAB REPUBLIC
Yellow fever
Country requirement: a yellow fever vaccination certificate is required from travellers over 6 months of age arriving from countries with risk of yellow fever transmission.

Yellow fever vaccine recommendation: no

Malaria: Very limited malaria risk due exclusively to *P. vivax* may exist from May to October inclusive in foci along the northern border, especially in rural areas of El Hasaka Governorate (no indigenous cases reported since 2005).

Recommended prevention: **none**

TAJIKISTAN
Yellow fever
Country requirement: no
Yellow fever vaccine recommendation: no

Malaria: Malaria risk due predominantly to *P. vivax* exists from June to October inclusive, particularly in southern areas (Khatlon Region), and in some central (Dushanbe), western (Gorno-Badakhshan), and northern (Leninabad Region) areas. *P. falciparum* resistant to chloroquine and sulfadoxine–pyrimethamine reported in the southern part of the country.

Recommended prevention in risk areas: **III**

TANZANIA, UNITED REPUBLIC OF, *see* UNITED REPUBLIC OF TANZANIA

THAILAND
Yellow fever
Country requirement: a yellow fever vaccination certificate is required from travellers over 9 months of age arriving from countries with risk of yellow fever transmission.

Yellow fever vaccine recommendation: no

Malaria: Malaria risk exists throughout the year in rural, especially forested and hilly, areas of the whole country, mainly towards the international borders, including the southernmost provinces. There is no risk in cities (e.g. Bangkok, Chiang Mai city, Pattaya), Samui island and the main tourist resorts of Phuket island. However, there is a risk in some other areas and islands. *P. falciparum* resistant to chloroquine and sulfadoxine–pyrimethamine reported. Resistance to mefloquine and to quinine reported from areas near the borders with Cambodia and Myanmar. *P. vivax* resistance to chloroquine reported. Human *P. knowlesi* infection reported.

Recommended prevention in risk areas: **I**; in areas near Cambodia and Myanmar borders: **IV**

THE FORMER YUGOSLAV REPUBLIC OF MACEDONIA
Yellow fever
Country requirement: no
Yellow fever vaccine recommendation: no

TIMOR-LESTE
Yellow fever
Country requirement: a yellow fever vaccination certificate is required from travellers over 1 year of age arriving from countries with risk of yellow fever transmission.

Yellow fever vaccine recommendation: no

Malaria: Malaria risk due predominantly to *P. falciparum* exists throughout the year in the whole country. *P. falciparum* resistant to chloroquine and sulfadoxine–pyrimethamine reported.

Recommended prevention: **IV**

TOGO
Yellow fever
Country requirement: a yellow fever vaccination certificate is required from all travellers over 1 year of age.

Yellow fever vaccine recommendation: yes

Malaria: Malaria risk due predominantly to *P. falciparum* exists throughout the year in the whole country. Chloroquine-resistant *P. falciparum* reported.

Recommended prevention: **IV**

228

TOKELAU

(Non-self-governing territory of New Zealand)

Same requirements as New Zealand.

TONGA

Yellow fever

Country requirement: no

Yellow fever vaccine recommendation: no

TRINIDAD AND TOBAGO

Yellow fever

Country requirement: a yellow fever vaccination certificate is required from travellers over 1 year of age arriving from countries with risk of yellow fever transmission.

Yellow fever vaccine recommendation: yes

Recommended for all travellers aged 9 months or over travelling to the island of Trinidad, except as mentioned below.

Generally not recommended[1] for travellers whose itineraries are limited to the urban areas of the Port of Spain, cruise ship passengers who do not disembark from the ship, and aeroplane passengers in transit.

Not recommended for travellers whose itineraries are limited to the island of Tobago.

TUNISIA

Yellow fever

Country requirement: a yellow fever vaccination certificate is required from travellers over 1 year of age arriving from countries with risk of yellow fever transmission.

Yellow fever vaccine recommendation: no

TURKEY

Yellow fever

Country requirement: no

Yellow fever vaccine recommendation: no

Malaria: Limited malaria risk due exclusively to *P. vivax* exists from May to October inclusive in

the south-eastern part of the country. There is no malaria risk in the main tourist areas in the west and south-west of the country.

Recommended prevention in risk areas: **II**

TURKMENISTAN

Yellow fever

Country requirement: no

Yellow fever vaccine recommendation: no

TUVALU

Yellow fever

Country requirement: no

Yellow fever vaccine recommendation: no

UGANDA

Yellow fever

Country requirement: a yellow fever vaccination certificate is required from travellers over 1 year of age arriving from countries with risk of yellow fever transmission.

Yellow fever vaccine recommendation: yes

Malaria: Malaria risk due predominantly to *P. falciparum* exists throughout the year in the whole country, including the main towns of Fort Portal, Jinja, Kampala, Kigezi and Mbale. Resistance to chloroquine and sulfadoxine–pyrimethamine reported.

Recommended prevention: **IV**

UKRAINE

Yellow fever

Country requirement: no

Yellow fever vaccine recommendation: no

UNITED ARAB EMIRATES

Yellow fever

Country requirement: no

Yellow fever vaccine recommendation: no

UNITED REPUBLIC OF TANZANIA

Yellow fever

Country requirement: a yellow fever vaccination certificate is required from travellers over 1 year of age arriving from countries with risk of yellow fever transmission.

---

[1] Yellow fever vaccination is *generally not recommended* in areas where there is low potential for exposure to yellow fever virus. However, vaccination might be considered for a small subset of travellers to these areas, who are at increased risk of exposure to yellow fever virus (e.g. prolonged travel, extensive exposure to mosquitoes, inability to avoid mosquito bites). When considering vaccination, any traveller must take into account the risk of being infected with yellow fever virus, country entry requirements, as well as individual risk factors (e.g. age, immune status) for serious vaccine-associated adverse events.

Yellow fever vaccine recommendation: in general, no:

Generally not recommended[1] for travellers to United Republic of Tanzania.

Malaria: Malaria risk due predominantly to *P. falciparum* exists throughout the year in the whole country below 1800 m. Resistance to chloroquine and sulfadoxine–pyrimethamine reported.

Recommended prevention in risk areas: **IV**

UNITED KINGDOM (WITH CHANNEL ISLANDS AND ISLE OF MAN)

Yellow fever

Country requirement: no

Yellow fever vaccine recommendation: no

UNITED STATES OF AMERICA

Yellow fever

Country requirement: no

Yellow fever vaccine recommendation: no

URUGUAY

Yellow fever

Country requirement: a yellow fever vaccination certificate is required from travellers arriving from countries with risk of yellow fever transmission.

Yellow fever vaccine recommendation: no

UZBEKISTAN

Yellow fever

Country requirement: no

Yellow fever vaccine recommendation: no

Malaria: Limited malaria risk due exclusively to *P. vivax* exists from June to October inclusive in some villages located in the southern and eastern parts of the country bordering Afghanistan, Kyrgyzstan and Tajikistan.

Recommended prevention in risk areas: **I**

---

[1] Yellow fever vaccination is *generally not recommended* in areas where there is low potential for exposure to yellow fever virus. However, vaccination might be considered for a small subset of travellers to these areas, who are at increased risk of exposure to yellow fever virus (e.g. prolonged travel, extensive exposure to mosquitoes, inability to avoid mosquito bites). When considering vaccination, any traveller must take into account the risk of being infected with yellow fever virus, country entry requirements, as well as individual risk factors (e.g. age, immune status) for serious vaccine-associated adverse events.

VANUATU

Yellow fever

Country requirement: no

Yellow fever vaccine recommendation: no

Malaria: Low to moderate malaria risk due predominantly to *P. falciparum* exists throughout the year in the whole country. *P. falciparum* resistant to chloroquine and sulfadoxine–pyrimethamine reported. *P. vivax* resistant to chloroquine reported.

Recommended prevention: **IV**

VENEZUELA (BOLIVARIAN REPUBLIC OF)

Yellow fever

Country requirement: no.

Yellow fever vaccine recommendation: yes

Recommended for all travellers aged 9 months or over, except as mentioned below.

Generally not recommended[1] for travellers whose itineraries are limited to the following areas: the entire states of Aragua, Carabobo, Miranda, Vargas and Yaracuy, and the Distrito Federal (Map).

Not recommended for travellers whose itineraries are limited to the following areas: the entire states of Falcon and Lara, the peninsular section of the Paez municipality of Zuila Province, Margarita Island, and the cities of Caracas and Valencia (Map).

Malaria: Malaria risk due to *P. vivax* (75%) and *P. falciparum* (25%) is moderate to high throughout the year in some rural areas of Amazonas, Anzoátegui, Bolívar and Delta Amacuro states. There is low risk in Apure, Monagas, Sucre and Zulia. Risk of *P. falciparum* malaria is mostly restricted to municipalities in jungle areas of Amazonas (Alto Orinoco, Atabapo, Atures, Autana, Manapiare) and Bolívar (Cedeño, El Callao, Heres, Gran Sabana, Piar, Raul Leoni, Rocio, Sifontes and Sucre). *P. falciparum* resistant to chloroquine and sulfadoxine–pyrimethamine reported.

Recommended prevention: **II** in *P. vivax* risk areas; **IV** in *P. falciparum* risk areas

VIET NAM

Yellow fever

Country requirement: a yellow fever vaccination certificate is required from travellers over 1 year of age arriving from countries with risk of yellow fever transmission.

Yellow fever vaccine recommendation: no

Malaria: Malaria risk due predominantly to *P. falciparum* exists in the whole country, excluding urban centres, the Red River delta, the Mekong delta, and the coastal plain areas of central Viet Nam. High-risk areas are the highland areas below 1500 m south of 18°N, notably in the four central highlands provinces Dak Lak, Dak Nong, Gia Lai and Kon Tum, Binh Phuoc province, and the western parts of the coastal provinces Khanh Hoa, Ninh Thuan, Quang Nam and Quang Tri. Resistance to chloroquine, sulfadoxine–pyrimethamine and mefloquine reported.

Recommended prevention in risk areas: **IV**

VIRGIN ISLANDS (USA)

Yellow fever

Country requirement: no

Yellow fever vaccine recommendation: no

WAKE ISLAND

(US territory)

Yellow fever

Country requirement: no

Yellow fever vaccine recommendation: no

YEMEN

Yellow fever

Country requirement: a yellow fever vaccination certificate is required from travellers over 1 year of age arriving from countries with risk of yellow fever transmission.

Yellow fever vaccine recommendation: no

Malaria: Malaria risk due predominantly to *P. falciparum* exists throughout the year, but mainly from September to February inclusive, in the whole country below 2000 m. There is no risk in Sana'a city. Malaria risk on Socotra Island

is very limited. Resistance to chloroquine and sulfadoxine–pyrimethamine reported.

Recommended prevention in risk areas: **IV**; Socotra Island: **I**

ZAIRE *see* DEMOCRATIC REPUBLIC OF THE CONGO

ZAMBIA

Yellow fever

Country requirement: no

Yellow fever vaccine recommendation: in general, no

Generally not recommended[1] for travellers going to the following areas: the entire North West and Western provinces

Not recommended in all other areas not listed above.

Malaria: Malaria risk due predominantly to *P. falciparum* exists throughout the year in the whole country, including Lusaka. Resistance to chloroquine and sulfadoxine–pyrimethamine reported.

Recommended prevention: **IV**

ZIMBABWE

Yellow fever

Country requirement: a yellow fever vaccination certificate is required from travellers arriving from countries with risk of yellow fever transmission.

Yellow fever vaccine recommendation: no

Malaria: Malaria risk due predominantly to *P. falciparum* exists from November to June inclusive in areas below 1200 m and throughout the year in the Zambezi valley. In Bulawayo and Harare, the risk is negligible. Resistance to chloroquine and sulfadoxine–pyrimethamine reported.

Recommended prevention in risk areas: **IV**

---

[1] Yellow fever vaccination is *generally not recommended* in areas where there is low potential for exposure to yellow fever virus. However, vaccination might be considered for a small subset of travellers to these areas, who are at increased risk of exposure to yellow fever virus (e.g. prolonged travel, extensive exposure to mosquitoes, inability to avoid mosquito bites). When considering vaccination, any traveller must take into account the risk of being infected with yellow fever virus, country entry requirements, as well as individual risk factors (e.g. age, immune status) for serious vaccine-associated adverse events.

Countries[1] with risk of yellow fever transmission[2] and countries requiring yellow fever vaccination

Countries	Countries with risk of yellow fever transmission	Countries requiring yellow fever vaccination for travellers arriving from countries with risk of yellow fever transmission	Countries requiring yellow fever vaccination for travellers from all countries
Afghanistan		Yes	
Albania		Yes	
Algeria		Yes	
Angola	Yes		Yes
Anguilla		Yes	
Antigua and Barbuda		Yes	
Argentina	Yes		
Australia		Yes	
Bahamas		Yes	
Bahrain		Yes	
Bangladesh		Yes	

---

[1] For the purpose of this publication, the terms "country" and "countries" cover countries, territories and areas.

[2] Risk of yellow fever transmission is defined as yellow fever being currently reported or having been reported in the past and presence of vectors and animal reservoirs representing a potential risk of infection and transmission. In the 2011 edition of *International Travel and Health*, Sao Tome and Principe, the United Republic of Tanzania as well as selected areas of Eritrea, Somalia and Zambia were reclassified as "areas with low potential for exposure" for yellow fever (see Country list).

Countries	Countries with risk of yellow fever transmission	Countries requiring yellow fever vaccination for travellers arriving from countries with risk of yellow fever transmission	Countries requiring yellow fever vaccination for travellers from all countries
Barbados		Yes	
Belize		Yes	
Benin	Yes		Yes
Bhutan		Yes	
Bolivia, Plurinational State of	Yes	Yes	
Botswana		Yes	
Brazil	Yes		
Brunei Darussalam		Yes	
Burkina Faso	Yes		Yes
Burundi	Yes		Yes
Cambodia		Yes	
Cameroon	Yes		Yes
Cape Verde		Yes	
Central African Republic	Yes		Yes
Chad	Yes	Yes	
China		Yes	
Christmas Island		Yes	
Colombia	Yes		
Congo	Yes		Yes
Costa Rica		Yes	
Côte d'Ivoire	Yes		Yes
Democratic People's Republic of Korea		Yes	
Democratic Republic of the Congo	Yes		Yes

Countries	Countries with risk of yellow fever transmission	Countries requiring yellow fever vaccination for travellers arriving from countries with risk of yellow fever transmission	Countries requiring yellow fever vaccination for travellers from all countries
Djibouti		Yes	
Dominica		Yes	
Ecuador	Yes	Yes	
Egypt		Yes	
El Salvador		Yes	
Equatorial Guinea	Yes	Yes	
Eritrea		Yes	
Ethiopia	Yes	Yes	
Fiji		Yes	
French Guiana	Yes		Yes
Gabon	Yes		Yes
Gambia	Yes	Yes	
Ghana	Yes		Yes
Grenada		Yes	
Guadeloupe		Yes	
Guatemala		Yes	
Guinea	Yes	Yes	
Guinea-Bissau	Yes		Yes
Guyana	Yes	Yes	
Haiti		Yes	
Honduras		Yes	
India		Yes	
Indonesia		Yes	
Iran (Islamic Republic of)		Yes	

Countries	Countries with risk of yellow fever transmission	Countries requiring yellow fever vaccination for travellers arriving from countries with risk of yellow fever transmission	Countries requiring yellow fever vaccination for travellers from all countries
Iraq		Yes	
Jamaica		Yes	
Jordan		Yes	
Kazakhstan		Yes	
Kenya	Yes	Yes	
Kiribati		Yes	
Lao People's Democratic Republic		Yes	
Lebanon		Yes	
Lesotho		Yes	
Liberia	Yes		Yes
Libyan Arab Jamahiriya		Yes	
Madagascar		Yes	
Malawi		Yes	
Malaysia		Yes	
Maldives		Yes	
Mali	Yes		Yes
Malta		Yes	
Martinique		Yes	
Mauritania	Yes	Yes	
Mauritius		Yes	
Montserrat		Yes	
Mozambique		Yes	
Myanmar		Yes	

Countries	Countries with risk of yellow fever transmission	Countries requiring yellow fever vaccination for travellers arriving from countries with risk of yellow fever transmission	Countries requiring yellow fever vaccination for travellers from all countries
Namibia		Yes	
Nauru		Yes	
Nepal		Yes	
Netherlands Antilles		Yes	
New Caledonia		Yes	
Nicaragua		Yes	
Niger	Yes		Yes
Nigeria	Yes	Yes	
Niue		Yes	
Oman		Yes	
Pakistan		Yes	
Panama	Yes	Yes	
Papua New Guinea		Yes	
Paraguay	Yes	Yes	
Peru	Yes		
Philippines		Yes	
Pitcairn Islands		Yes	
Reunion		Yes	
Russian Federation		Yes	
Rwanda	Yes		Yes
Saint Helena		Yes	
Saint Kitts and Nevis		Yes	
Saint Lucia		Yes	
Saint Vincent and the Grenadines		Yes	

Countries	Countries with risk of yellow fever transmission	Countries requiring yellow fever vaccination for travellers arriving from countries with risk of yellow fever transmission	Countries requiring yellow fever vaccination for travellers from all countries
Samoa		Yes	
Sao Tome and Principe			Yes
Saudi Arabia		Yes	
Senegal	Yes	Yes	
Seychelles		Yes	
Sierra Leone	Yes		Yes
Singapore		Yes	
Solomon Islands		Yes	
Somalia		Yes	
South Africa		Yes	
Sri Lanka		Yes	
Sudan	Yes	Yes	
Suriname	Yes	Yes	
Swaziland		Yes	
Syrian Arab Republic		Yes	
Thailand		Yes	
Timor Leste		Yes	
Togo	Yes		Yes
Trinidad and Tobago	Yes (Trinidad only)	Yes	
Tunisia		Yes	
Uganda	Yes	Yes	
United Republic of Tanzania		Yes	
Uruguay		Yes	

Countries	Countries with risk of yellow fever transmission	Countries requiring yellow fever vaccination for travellers arriving from countries with risk of yellow fever transmission	Countries requiring yellow fever vaccination for travellers from all countries
Venezuela (Bolivarian Republic of)	Yes		
Viet Nam		Yes	
Yemen		Yes	
Zimbabwe		Yes	

International Health Regulations

The spread of infectious diseases from one part of the world to another is not a new phenomenon, but in recent decades a number of factors have underscored the fact that infectious disease events in one country may be of potential concern for the entire world. These factors include: increased population movements, whether through tourism or migration or as a result of disasters; growth in international trade in food; biological, social and environmental changes linked with urbanization; deforestation; alterations in climate; and changes in methods of food processing, distribution and consumer habits. Consequently, the need for international cooperation in order to safeguard global health has become increasingly important.

The International Health Regulations (IHR), adopted in 1969, amended in 1973 and 1981[1] and completely revised in 2005,[2] provide the legal framework for such international cooperation. The stated purpose of the Regulations is to prevent, protect against, control, and provide public health responses to the international spread of disease in ways that are commensurate with and restricted to public health risks, and that avoid unnecessary interference with international traffic and trade.

Their main objectives are to ensure: (1) the appropriate application of routine preventive measures (e.g. at ports and airports) and the use by all countries of internationally approved documents (e.g. vaccination certificates); (2) the notification to WHO of all events that may constitute a public health emergency of international concern; and (3) the implementation of any temporary recommendations should the WHO Director-General determine that such an emergency is occurring. In addition to new notification and reporting requirements, the IHR (2005) focus on the provision of support for affected states and the avoidance of stigma and unnecessary negative impact on international travel and trade.

---

[1] *International Health Regulations (1969): third annotated edition.* Geneva, World Health Organization, 1983.

[2] *International Health Regulations (2005):* www.who.int/ihr

The IHR (2005) entered into force on 15 June 2007. They take account of the present volume of international traffic and trade and of current trends in the epidemiology of infectious diseases, as well as other emerging and re-emerging health risks.

The two specific applications of the IHR (2005) most likely to be encountered by travellers are the yellow fever vaccination requirements imposed by certain countries (see Chapter 6 and country list) and the disinsection of aircraft to prevent importation of disease vectors (see Chapter 2).[3]

The vaccination requirements and disinsection measures are intended to help prevent the international spread of diseases and, in the context of international travel, to do so with the minimum inconvenience to the traveller. This requires international collaboration in the detection and reduction or elimination of the sources of infection.

Ultimately, the risk of an infectious agent becoming established in a country is determined by the quality of the national epidemiological and public health capacities and, in particular, by day-to-day national health and disease surveillance activities and the ability to detect and implement prompt and effective control measures. The requirements for states to establish certain minimum capacities in this regard will, when implemented, provide increased security for visitors as well as for the resident population of the country.

---

[3] Hardiman M., Wilder-Smith A. The revised international health regulations and their relevance to the travel medicine practitioner. *Journal of Travel Medicine*, 2007, 14(3):141–144.

Index of countries and territories

Index by subject

First aid
  animal bites, 40–41, 114–119
  in-flight, 25
  kits, 25
  snake/scorpion/spider/bites, 41–42
Fish
  poisoning, 42
  venomous, 42–43
Fishing, 39, 53
Fleas, 45, 76
Flies bloodsucking, 44
Flight phobia, 20
Flotation aids, 38–39
Fluid intake
  air travellers, 6
  in hot climates, 33–34
  in travellers' diarrhoea, 36
  see also Drinks; Water
Flying *see* Air travel
Food
  -borne health risks, 36, 55
  hygiene, 2–3, 12, 36, 48, 55, 58–59, 93, 111, 126, 179, 181, 183, 185
  safety precautions, 36–37
Footwear, 16, 122
Frequent travellers, 5, 7, 10, 22, 28, 37, 44, 51, 60, 90–91, 135, 154, 195
Fruit, 47–48, 65, 126
Fungal skin infections, 34, 40

Gas expansion in-flight, 15–16
Gastroenteritis *see also* Travellers' diarrhoea
Genital herpes, 69–70
Genital warts, 69, 98
Giardiasis (*Giardia*) infections, 39–40, 65
Glucose-6-phosphate dehydrogenase (G6PD) deficiency, 152
Gonorrhoea, 69–70

Haemophilia, 169
Haemophilus influenzae type b Hib
  meningitis, 92
  vaccination, 84, 92
  vaccine, 84, 92
Haemorrhagic fever with renal syndrome (HFRS), 66
Haemorrhagic fevers, 45, 56, 65–66
HAI *see* High-altitude illness
Hajj pilgrims, 86, 105, 107, 134, 176–177, 184
Halofantrine, 161, 164

Hantavirus diseases, 66, 68
Hantavirus pulmonary syndrome (HPS), 66
Head injuries, 52–53
Heat
  exhaustion, 33–34, 38
  prickly, 34
Helminth infections intestinal, 46
Hepatitis chronic, 7, 68, 94
Hepatitis A
  geographical distribution, 68, 70–71, 93, 126
  immunoglobulin, 183
  vaccine
    adverse reactions, 94, 101, 177
    combinations, 84
    in pregnancy, 101, 136–137
Hepatitis B
  exposure to blood body fluids and, 96, 169–170, 173
  geographical distribution, 68–71, 93
  prophylaxis, 68–70, 93, 170, 172–174, 185
  transmission, 56, 68–69, 71, 92, 94, 96, 169–170, 177
  treatment, 70, 92, 137, 169, 172, 185
  vaccine
    adverse reactions, 94, 177
    combination, 84, 93, 96, 184
    in elderly, 136–137
    in pregnancy, 136–137
Hepatitis C, 56, 68, 140, 169–170, 172–173, 185
Hepatitis E, 6, 36, 68, 93, 135, 173
Herpes genital, 69–70
Hib *see Haemophilus influenzae* type b
High-altitude, 13, 32–33, 50
High-altitude cerebral oedema, 32
High-altitude illness, 32, 50
High-altitude pulmonary oedema, 32
Hijacking vehicle, 54
HIV/AIDS
  exposure to blood body fluids and, 96
  geographical distribution, 58, 69
  precautions, 58, 69, 82, 96, 98
  risk for travellers, 69, 98, 159, 177
  transmission, 56, 58, 69, 96, 98, 177
  treatment, 58, 159
  vaccination, 82, 98, 177
Hookworms, 47
Hormone-replacement therapy, 18
Human immunodeficiency virus *see* HIV